*Sugars That Heal* is a breakthrough book. Unfortunately, information about beneficial, healing sugars and polysaccharides has been "lost" in the well-deserved ocean of bad publicity about our nation's enormous overconsumption of sucrose, fructose, and refined carbohydrates. In *Sugars That Heal,* Dr. Emil Mondoa and Mindy Kitei present for us a well-documented book about the *good* sugars and polysaccharides, with details on both their preventive and therapeutic effects. This book will fill an important gap in our health libraries. Highly recommended!

—JONATHAN V. WRIGHT, M.D., coauthor of
*The Patient's Book of Natural Healing*
and *Natural Hormone Replacement*

# SUGARS
# THAT
# HEAL

**The New Healing Science of Glyconutrients**

EMIL I. MONDOA, M.D.
AND MINDY KITEI

THE BALLANTINE PUBLISHING GROUP | NEW YORK

This book is not intended as a substitute for medical advice. Consult your doctor before beginning any of the recommendations in this book and follow the precautions and caveats that the author has specified. Also, individual results achieved by following the recommendations in *Sugars That Heal* may vary, depending on each person's unique attributes and the severity of his or her disease. WARNING: No pregnant or nursing woman should take any glyconutrient supplements.

A Ballantine Book
Published by The Ballantine Publishing Group
Copyright © 2001 Emil I. Mondoa, M.D., and Mindy Kitei

www.ballantinebooks.com

Library of Congress Cataloging-in-Publication Data
Mondoa, Emil I.
Sugars that heal : the new healing science of glyconutrients /
by Emil I. Mondoa and Mindy Kitiei.—1st ed.
p.     cm.
Includes bibliographical references and index.
1. Sugars—Health aspects. 2. Sugars—Therapeutic use. I. Kitei, Mindy.
II. Title.
QP702.S85 M66 2001
612.3'96—dc21          2001035219

ISBN 0-345-44106-0

Manufactured in the United States of America

First Edition: August 2001

10  9  8  7  6  5  4  3

*To my mother, Susannah N. Mondoa*
—EM

*To my dad, Milton N. Kitei, M.D.*
—MK

# Contents

- A hundred years ago, Harvard-educated physician William Coley figured out that saccharides, the scientific word for sugars, could cure certain cancers.
- Glyconutrients are the foods and supplements that contain essential saccharides.
- Multicellular intelligence: How saccharides mediate the body's communication and healing capabilities.

# Acknowledgments

Many people contributed to making this book a reality, and we appreciate all those who took the time to help us. We are indebted to Paul Hoskin, Blair Davis, and Terry Murray for their excellent research. Thanks to all those who shared their personal stories, to Tom Starner for cheerfully fixing the computers, to Abby Durden at Ballantine, and, most especially, to Leslie Meredith, our editor at Ballantine, for her exceptional counsel and enduring faith.

Emil would like to thank his wife, Ambrosia, and daughter Matanda for their support and confidence during the painstaking book-writing process. Friends and colleagues provided tremendous support as well. Professor Victor Anomah Ngu provided inspiration, while Dr. Tayoba Ngenge furnished sage advice. Emil is also grateful for the help provided by Dr. Bernard Jiburum, Dr. Yoshimi Shibata, Fred Kafes, Edward Dilingian, Janelle Leatherwood, Dr. Everett Nichols, Dr. Carlton Turner,

Dr. H. Reg McDaniel, Lori Siegler, Dr. Isaac Elias, Deborah Caplow, Dr. Georges Halpern, and Jane D. Saxton. Special thanks go to Emil's literary agent, Jeremy Solomon of First Books.

Mindy would like to thank her father, Dr. Milton Kitei, brother Dr. Robert Kitei, sister-in-law Georganne Kitei, cousin Lisa Kitei, lawyer Bob Solomon at Frankfort Garbus, and Jeremy Solomon for their astute advice and support. To Lou Harry, Cindy Weiss Harry, Ward Karns, Louis Massiah, Tracey Diehl, Kevin Diehl, Ronnie Polaneczky, Noel Weyrich, Patti Schmidt, David Schmidt, Nancy Kaiser, Jim Kaiser, Sandra Soll, Pat Cope, Allen Rubin, Robin Switzenbaum, and Tim Haas go her thanks for their unflagging good humor. She's especially grateful to long-time friend and indefatigable editor Larry Closs, and to Rhea and Arielle, who never tired of asking, "Is it done yet?"

# Preface

*"Hope is a good thing, probably the best of things. . . ."*
—Andy (Tim Robbins) in a letter to Red (Morgan Freeman)
  in the movie *The Shawshank Redemption*

I first tried essential saccharides, the scientific term for sugars, in the fall of 1996. By that time, I was at the lowest point of a difficult five-year period in my life. My father had died the year before on Christmas Eve, and I was working 80 to 100 hours a week at different hospitals, mostly during weekends and at night. In the daytime, I was pursuing my MBA in health care at the Wharton School of the University of Pennsylvania, having completed my residency in pediatrics at the Medical Center of Delaware. During that time our daughter, Matanda, was born very prematurely, which increased the worry and stress on us all. (We are blessed because she has done extremely well.) The topper was that my immigration status in the United States was under review, and my wife and I weren't sure that I'd be allowed to complete my Wharton degree.

I had reached my breaking point, and my usually good health was deteriorating. Exhausted, I had frequent colds and began to experience chest pain. My father and his father before him had died of heart attacks, so I was concerned. And then a red, scaly rash appeared and began inching up my thighs to my torso, toward my neck and face. Dermatology and infectious-disease colleagues thought it was a fungal infection, but the rash didn't respond to antifungal medications and responded only temporarily to steroid creams.

I decided to take matters into my own hands and trust my instincts. I began to watch my diet more closely and to exercise more. Like many physicians, I didn't then believe that nutritional supplements did any good, but I was worried enough to hedge my bets by taking daily multivitamins. Having grown up in a culture in what was then the Southern Cameroons, Africa, where most of the food was organic and eaten freshly picked, I had never really gotten used to the American diet based on industrially grown food, so I began to eat more natural, less processed foods again. While I felt better changing my diet and exercising more, the rash was as fiery as ever. A serendipitous call from a former colleague at the Wharton School who had become interested in saccharides and glyconutrients—the foods and supplements that contain the essential saccharides—changed things.

At my friend's suggestion, I started reading up on saccharides, and what struck me was the influence of essential sugars in practically all functions of the human body, particularly in helping to regulate the immune system. So I decided to try them; I figured I had nothing to lose. I purchased a small tub of Ambrotose, a powder that contains the eight essential saccharides. (See the resources section for more information on this and other products.) I took one gram daily (that's 1,000 milligrams) in divided doses, morning and evening. Within a week I felt calmer and more energetic. I was hopeful but also considered that the improvement might be a placebo effect, that it was my expectations of getting well rather than the saccharides that were helping. Usually placebo responses are relatively short-lived. But if it was a placebo response, it has lasted four years: the rash that had plagued me for more than six months regressed and disappeared completely in a month's time, never to return. My chest pain resolved as well. I was so enthusiastic I contacted Mannatech, the company whose product I was using, and went on to serve as a consultant for a few years, all the while acquiring more knowledge about saccharides and glyconutrients on my own. Much of the information came from reading studies from China and Japan, for the simple reason that these countries have conducted by far the most saccharide trials.

In the years since I started on glyconutrients—the foods and supplements that contain essential saccharides—I've been well, except for two relatively mild colds. My wife, Ambrosia, takes them, too, and she has noted an increase in energy that began about two months into glyconutritional supplementation with Ambrotose. My entire family has tried several different kinds of glyconutrients by different manufacturers, many of which are listed in the resources section, and has had good experiences with them. We've also added shiitake mushrooms, an excellent source of essential saccharides, to our diets. In addition, I take two grams of an extract from a Chinese mushroom called cordyceps daily in divided doses. Occasionally, when I'm stressed, I add a 250-milligram capsule of a glyconutrient extract called a beta-glucan, which in this case is made from yeast. (Other beta-glucans come from rice, barley, oats, and mushrooms.)

Since my own experience, I've suggested to several of my patients that they try glyconutrients. I have seen good results in patients for whom medications like antibiotics and steroids hadn't worked. Glyconutrients have also helped patients for whom medications such as antibiotics and steroids worked well—temporarily. After the drugs were withdrawn, the patients' problems returned with a vengeance, but sometimes glyconutrients arrested the problem where traditional medications could not.

While glyconutrients are natural substances that come from foods, they are not right for everyone. One to 2 percent of the population is allergic to any particular food—and glyconutrients are no exception. If you are allergic to mushrooms, for instance, you must avoid glyconutrient mushrooms or extracts from mushrooms. In addition, some extracts, pectins, and mush-rooms contain substances that thin the blood. If you have bleed-ing problems or take medications that thin the blood (including Coumadin, heparin, Plavix, Motrin, Naprosyn, Vioxx, Celebrex, Mobic, ibuprofen, or aspirin), consult your doctor before start-ing glyconutrients and mushrooms or mushroom-derived prod-ucts and read the dos and don'ts of taking glyconutrients in chapter 3.

Glyconutrients have a role in preventing some illnesses and helping induce recovery from others, including cancer, autoim-mune diseases, neurological disorders, and chronic or recurrent infections. In some cases, glyconutrients awaken the immune sys-tem as if from a coma and the body begins to respond, naturally fighting off pathogens more effectively—as it should have done in the first place—without any harmful effects. The gentleness of glyconutrients' actions stands in stark contrast with the harsh side effects of the many powerful drugs we use today to treat seri-ous disease. Virtually any medication has side effects—physicians and researchers routinely uncover new and unsuspected ones. Natural substances—including foods—have side effects, too, but they are usually less problematic because, unlike drugs, natural substances are less concentrated.

In the future, medicine will be a more tender art, bearing little resemblance to today's martial treatments, with more em-phasis on prevention. I believe that glyconutrients will play a sig-nificant role in shifting the focus in health care from treatment to prevention. Even now, glyconutrients can significantly help to keep you well. They can also be a complement to your own doc-tor's recommendations for treating certain illnesses you may have—although you must *always consult* with your doctor before starting to take glyconutrients if you are already taking drugs your doctor has prescribed, or over-the-counter blood thinners like aspirin or ibuprofen.

As this book will show, saccharides are essential in virtually all intelligent interactions between the cells of the body; they're a crucial part of cell intelligence and activity. Glyconutrients affect how our cells form the structure of the body and the daily repair of our tissues. They play an important role in helping our body distinguish what belongs in it from what does not belong, and so they are vital to how our cells react to bacteria and viruses. Of course, if someone is undernourished, glyconutrients will provide little or no defense. You need to have a healthy diet for any supplement to work optimally.

A healthy diet and lifestyle help to maintain, restore, and optimize the body and its functions. Yet because the pharmaceutical industry doesn't devote much attention or money to natural substances and foods that can't be patented, nutrition is not a big part of the business of medicine. Nevertheless, over the past decade interest in natural health, and glyconutrients in particular, has increased and many studies have been conducted. Scientists have concluded in many cases that the effects of glyconutrients on both healthy people and those patients with serious, chronic medical conditions have been significant.

For instance, researchers have discovered that glucosamine, a metabolic product of the essential saccharide N-acetylglucosamine, is an effective treatment for a common form of arthritis known as osteoarthritis. (See chapter 10 for more information.) First used by veterinarians to treat arthritis in dogs, cats, and horses, glucosamine became a popular treatment for people with arthritic knees in the mid 1990s. According to a 2001 study published in the prestigious journal *Lancet*, scientists found that glucosamine not only relieved the pain and inflammation caused by the disease but also *reversed* damage by rebuilding cartilage that gets worn away as the arthritis progresses. In fact, glucosamine and a complex sugar called chondroitin are the only known substances that repair cartilage damage.

Other glyconutrients have equally impressive healing effects. *Sugars That Heal* presents exciting new scientific findings on these glyconutrients. It sheds light on how they help optimize the workings of the immune and nervous systems to boost the body's innate powers of healing. *Sugars That Heal* also introduces you to the nutritional sources of the essential saccharides in foods and supplements, and offers practical ways for you to use them to help maintain or improve your health.

If you already have one of the conditions covered in the book, discuss with your doctor how to use glyconutrients to complement your current medical treatments. Your physician can help chart a course for you to stay healthy or heal, but it is your job to stay that course. The responsibility for improving your health is primarily in your own hands: what happens on a daily basis *outside* your doctor's office is just as important—if not more so—than what happens *inside* the doctor's office. Only you can assume responsibility for taking your medication and sticking to a diet or exercise program. Knowledge is power, and knowledge about glyconutrients—a kinder, gentler, natural healing agent—can empower you to get and stay healthy.

# PART I

# WHAT ARE SACCHARIDES AND WHY ARE THEY IMPORTANT?

"It is not . . . that some people do not know what to do with truth when it is offered them, but the tragic fate is to reach, after patient search, a condition of mind-blindness, in which the truth is not recognized, though it stares you in the face."
—*Sir William Osler, physician, 1849–1919*

## Chapter 1

# Coley's Saccharides

*Though he didn't know why they worked, more than a hundred years ago a Harvard-educated physician named William Coley figured out that saccharides could cure certain cancers.*

In the fall of 1890, Elizabeth Dashiell, a delicate young woman of seventeen, was diagnosed with bone cancer in her right hand. Since her diagnosis had come early in the course of the disease, amputation of her afflicted arm below the elbow was swift. Yet she died a few months later. Her doctor, twenty-eight-year-old Harvard Medical School graduate William Coley, was distraught. A surgeon at New York's Memorial Hospital, which would later be renamed Memorial Sloan-Kettering Cancer Center, Coley began poring over old patient records—for what, he wasn't sure. As Coley read the dusty charts, he saw that most cancer therapies failed; most of the patients died. But curiously, one patient who was severely afflicted with sarcoma, a cancer of the connective tissue, did recuperate.[1, 2] Hospitalized and near death in the fall of 1884, he experienced two outbreaks of a severe skin infection called erysipelas. Caused by a strep bacterium, the infections resulted in high fevers and roused his immune system. The bumpy, plum-sized tumor below his left ear began to shrink and the patient rallied, recovering completely. When the tenacious Coley tracked the man down, he was well, with no cancer recurrence some seven years later.

Because Coley's discovery transpired more than a century ago when the immune system was uncharted territory, the scientist didn't understand how the patient's strep infection could bring about a cancer remission. Nevertheless, the prescient physician thought perhaps he had stumbled across something important— a novel way to treat cancer—and began a series of experiments on sarcoma patients.[3] Coley's quest to reproduce what nature had so elegantly accomplished is detailed with heart-thumping vigor by writer Stephen Hall in his excellent book *A Commotion in the Blood*.[4] According to Hall, after repeated failures in inoculating a sarcoma patient with live cultures of the strep bacterium, Coley eventually procured an exceptionally potent strain that induced a high fever and skin infection in the lucky man who received it. Within a few weeks the patient's neck tumors began to recede, eventually vanished, and didn't return for several years—and the young surgeon soon published his first paper.

Using live, virulent bacteria was, naturally, dangerous (in fact, two of Coley's patients died from resulting strep infections), so the doctor eventually developed a safer method, devising a vaccine. After culturing the bacteria, Coley killed the colonies or filtered them out, his theory being that the toxins the cultured bacteria had produced were at least partly responsible for the tumor shrinkage.[5] In due course, Coley added the toxins from a second bacterium, which today is called *Serratia marcescens*. That combination proved remarkably successful. On advanced, inoperable sarcomas he accomplished a cure rate of close to 20 percent with his treatment. When the toxin therapy was continued for six months after surgery, Coley's five-year remission rates soared to 80 percent, according to a retrospective study done by Coley's daughter.[6] That figure rivals, and in some cases surpasses, current sarcoma treatment outcomes, without the long-term consequences of today's chemotherapies and radiation.

For a short time, Coley's toxins—also known as fever therapy because the treatment induced high fevers—was the only recognized systemic treatment for cancer other than surgery. Coley's crude bacterial immunotherapy, however, was never really accepted in scientific circles. Quality control was one reason. The toxins weren't standardized, nor was the dosing, and many physicians with inferior batches didn't get good results.[7, 8] In addition, vaccine therapy wasn't a top priority for pharmaceutical companies. There wasn't then, and there isn't now, much money in it. And since turn-of-the century medicine had no understanding of the immune system, scientists lacked the framework for understanding why the toxins worked.[9] The final demise of toxin therapy came with the advent of radiation therapy.

At first, physicians often used the two therapies together. But as writer Stephen Hall explains, radiation became so fashionable that Coley's overzealous boss, the then-head of Memorial Hospital, Dr. James Ewing, advised his staff to use high-dose radiation not only for bone cancer but also for all instances of "persistent unexplained" bone pain.[10] Meanwhile, Coley's toxins became yesterday's news, even though the treatment appeared to work better than radiation. Of twenty-four patients with inoperable sarcoma at Memorial Hospital treated with radiation alone, twenty-one were dead and the other three had had treatment too recent to evaluate.[11] In contrast, of twenty-two inoperable sarcoma cases treated with Coley's toxins, some in conjunction with radiation, some not, twelve patients remained cancer-free after five years, the benchmark for a clinical cure.[12]

Damn the statistics—radium was, in a word, hot, and Coley's toxins were not. Like lambs to the slaughter, the unsuspecting public joined the radium craze on an unregulated, recreational level. Dubbed "mild radium therapy" to distinguish it from the high radium levels reserved for cancer treatment, over-the-counter radium-enhanced products became de rigueur.[13] Radium foot salves were up-to-the-minute at the turn of the century; for men only, a radium-fortified jockstrap was available. Manufacturers laced candy with radium and spiked designer water called Radithor with it, touting the one-dollar-a-bottle brew as an energy elixir for 150 "endocrinologic" ailments, from rheumatism and hypertension to exhaustion and sexual dysfunction.[14, 15] Indeed, the doctor's pamphlet that accompanied Radithor boasted that its "tonic effects upon the nervous system generally result in a great improvement in the sex organs."[16] Not surprisingly, more than 400,000 bottles were sold.

Recreational radium finally lost its luster soon after forty-seven-year-old Pittsburgh playboy, steel tycoon and former amateur golf champion Eben M. Byers, on his doctor's advice, began imbibing Radithor daily to nurse an arm injury. Invigorated, he tripled his dose but gradually began feeling tired and losing weight. By the time he figured out why, it was too late. The toothless Food and Drug Administration(FDA) at the time could only issue warnings. Not so for the Federal Trade Commission(FTC). In a surreal twist, the FTC at first took action against those radium elixirs that *failed* to meet their advertised levels of radium.[17]

As for Byers, the radium had dissolved much of his upper and lower jaws in short order and bored holes in his skull, causing pain and disfigurement. "The Radium Water Worked Fine Until His Jaw Came Off" proclaimed the blunt *Wall Street Journal* headline, curtly summing up Eben Byers's disastrous experience with Radithor.[18] The once rakish, robust industrialist was a time-worn, shrunken 92 pounds fading into the starched white sheets at Doctors' Hospital in New York City, where he died at age fifty-one on March 31, 1932, and made front-page news.[19] A few months before, the FTC had stepped in and put a stop to Radithor, and before long the FDA was regulating the chemical element.

Astonishingly, Byers's death didn't taint the use of high-dose radiation—perhaps because with Coley's toxins passé, there were no other cancer-treatment options at the time besides surgery. After Coley's death in 1936, his immunotherapy plunged from outré to oblivion.

Then, in 1943, a scientist at the National Cancer Institute (NCI) discovered that a lipopolysaccharide—a fat bonded to a saccharide, the scientific word for sugar—was the biologically active substance in the toxins of *Serratia marcescens*, one of the components of Coley's vaccine. In this case, the lipopolysaccharides resided in the cell walls of the *Serratia marcescens* bacteria. The fat in the lipopolysaccharide could cause toxicity problems, however; scientists eventually pared the fat from the sugar, leaving a nontoxic compound with salutary immune-system effects. These compounds incite the body to stimulate the immune cells and produce proteins called cytokines, which make you feel achy and fluish as they do battle with pathogens loitering in their path.[20, 21]

Unfortunately, the NCI discovery did nothing to resurrect the popularity of Coley's therapy. In fact, in 1965, in a mind-boggling move, the American Cancer Society added Coley's toxins to its list of "unproven" cancer drugs, in essence pronouncing his invention quackery, along with the likes of coffee enemas and laetrile.[22] Although the pronouncement was lifted ten years later, the bad publicity had sealed the fate of this undervalued treatment in the United States.

Vaccine therapy, however, remained popular in other countries. German scientists continued with their research, as did the Chinese. Bacterial vaccines have been most effective for sarcomas, lymphomas, and melanomas. Coley's vaccine has yielded impressive results, but thanks to one hundred years of scientific inertia, politics, and greed propagated by an unwitting confederacy of dunces, it's still not an established treatment for cancer. In all probability Coley's vaccine never will be because you can't patent a century-old drug.

Many discoveries of the first rank are for a time ignored or ridiculed. (Conversely, many discoveries, like radiation therapy, are for a time overrated.) What happened to the discovery of William Coley, who died largely forgotten and broke, having lost his money in the stock market crash of 1929, was, sadly, nothing new. What was new, though Coley didn't know it at the time, was that he made the first scientific association between the immune system and saccharides, the sugars that heal.

As an early indication of saccharides' worth, Coley's toxins are just the tip of the iceberg. In the past twenty years, the amount of information garnered about these sugars has increased dramatically. Of the more than two hundred sugars, eight are essential to optimal body functioning. Far more than just a ready source of fuel for the cells, these eight essential sugars have potent antiviral, antibacterial, antiparasitic, and of course antitumor effects.[23]

Essential saccharides have also been shown in clinical trials to reduce allergies and to allay symptoms in such chronic diseases as arthritis, diabetes, lupus, and kidney disease. They accelerate the healing of burns and wounds and help heal skin conditions—from poison ivy to psoriasis. They increase the body's resistance to viruses, including those that cause the common cold, influenza, herpes, and hepatitis. They quell the recurrent bacterial ear infections that plague toddlers and children. Some people with fibromyalgia, chronic fatigue syndrome, Gulf War syndrome, and HIV have reported improvement in their symptoms when they supplement their diet with these simple sugars.

## The Eight Essential Saccharides

When most of us think of sugar, we think only of table sugar from sugarcane, which consists of two saccharides, glucose and fructose. The eight essential saccharides our bodies need are mannose, glucose, galactose, xylose, fucose (not to be confused with fructose), N-acetylglucosamine, N-acetylgalactosamine, and N-acetylneuraminic acid. These eight essential saccharides compose the main focus of *Sugars That Heal.* Only two of these essential sugars, glucose (found in plants and table sugar) and galactose (found in milk products and certain pectins), are common in our diets. Although fructose, found in fruits and table sugar, is also a part of most diets, it's not an essential saccharide.

## What Are Glyconutrients?

The eight saccharides serve as the building blocks for the manufacture of large molecules made of sugars in combination with proteins and/or fats called *glycoforms*, which cover the surface of all cells. *Glycoproteins* are molecules made of sugars and proteins;

*glycolipids* are made of sugars and fats. *Glyconutrients* are the foods and nutritional supplements that provide the saccharides and glycoforms essential in our bodies but scarce in most of our diets. In Greek, glyco means "sweet"; *glyconutrient* literally means "sweet nutrient."

But some of these saccharides aren't sweet; some are tasteless, others bitter. All can be burned as energy. In the small quantities needed—for most people, the dose is half a teaspoon to a teaspoon of these sugars daily—they won't make you fat or raise your insulin levels, which can lead to diabetes down the road. In fact, they've been shown in studies to help you lose weight (see chapter 13); they're safe for diabetics and fit into low-carbohydrate diets.

Glyconutrients—the foods and nutritional supplements that provide saccharides—have powerful effects on the immune system. Glyconutrients can reactivate the immune system to shrink cancerous tumors and, in some cases, prevent or slow the progression of cancers in animals and humans. Even when the cancer has spread, or metastasized, glyconutrients have prolonged survival and improved quality of life. They have been found to be an effective adjunct when used in combination with surgery, chemotherapy, and radiation, both by mitigating the side effects of radiation and chemotherapy and by potentiating their cancer-killing effects.

Glyconutrients help the body heal. For instance, clinical trials have proved that glucosamine, a metabolic product of the essential saccharide N-acetylglucosamine, is effective in treating osteoarthritis, a common type of arthritis in older adults in which the cartilage around bone joints wears away, causing pain and swelling. Either alone or together with the polysaccharide chondroitin, glucosamine relieves pain and inflammation. In addition, studies confirm that the sugars help repair damaged cartilage—something ibuprofen and other traditional arthritis pain relievers can't do (see chapter 10 for more).

Glyconutrients and the saccharides that they provide also address the workings of the brain and nervous system—from memory and sleep to anxiety and depression. They have a role in helping people and animals handle cholesterol and fats properly, lowering triglycerides and low-density lipoproteins, or LDL (the so-called bad cholesterol), and raising high-density lipoproteins, or HDL (the "good" cholesterol). TV commercials tout the benefits of eating oatmeal to bring down cholesterol. But what the commercials don't say is that it's the sugars called betaglucans in the oatmeal that are responsible (see chapter 15).

Another important saccharide function is to help retain bone density and muscle mass, both of which diminish with age. As we live and move, our bodies undergo wear and tear. The cells and tissues of the body need to be replaced, remodeled, and renewed. When we modify our activity by, say, exercising, the body adapts. New blood vessels develop, muscles increase in mass. Certain kinds of tissues adapt by increasing the size and number of cells. Adaptation, healing, and recovery from wear and tear are all forms of tissue remodeling. Essential saccharides play important roles in such tissue resculpting.

The benefits of glyconutrients are so wide-ranging that they might appear unrelated to each other. On the one hand, it is rational to be skeptical that one group of substances could have such a broad range of benefits. (It slices, it dices, it makes julienne fries; it's a dessert topping and a floor polish!) On the other hand, it's intuitive that unifying factors and systems govern the apparent complexity of our bodies. The divisions that we place between systems and organs in our bodies are to an extent artificial and mostly for the convenience of our work and intellect. Our anatomy as we define it is a Western phenomenon. In China, unlike in the United States, the most highly regarded remedies are those that work for many illnesses; the least impressive are those that zero in on one disease. But the body itself doesn't rely on medical specialties to distinguish between its own parts—it is we who make artificial distinctions and develop medical specialties to deal with our more than two thousand body parts. To the body, however, all is one and one is all.

# The Power of One

*Monosaccharide* comes from the Greek *monos,* which means "one," and *sakcharon,* meaning "sugar." From monosaccharides—the simplest form of sugar—more complex molecules are assembled. Two saccharides link together to form a substance with two molecules called a *disaccharide.* Sucrose (from cane sugar and sugar beets) is a disaccharide, as is lactose. Found in milk, lactose consists of one molecule of glucose and one of galactose. *Oligosaccharides* consist of three to six monosaccharides and are found in breast milk and plants; they coat our mucus-membrane linings and are present in saliva. Link many monosaccharides together—from hundreds to thousands—and you fashion a very large molecule called a *polysaccharide.* Starch is a polysaccharide, as is glycogen. Stored in the liver as a backup source of fuel, our bodies convert glycogen back to glucose when we need the energy. The pages on which these words are written are composed of another polysaccharide called cellulose. Unlike other creatures, including deer that feast in your garden and termites that munch the clapboard on your house, we cannot digest cellulose because our guts do not possess the necessary enzyme.

The chemical structures of saccharides convey distinct, stable cellular messages. The saccharide molecule contains component atoms of carbon, hydrogen, and oxygen arranged in a ring. The ratio is always 1:2:1. So for every unit of carbon and oxygen there are two units of hydrogen. In the case of glucose, for instance, there are six carbon atoms, twelve hydrogen, and six oxygen.

The way in which the individual sugar molecules are joined to each other determines how the body absorbs and uses them. Consider a piece of coal and a diamond. It's hard to think of two objects more different from each other. Yet both are pure carbon. The difference lies in the way in which the individual atoms bond to each other. Likewise, the way the individual saccharide molecules of the eight essential saccharides bond to each other appears to be nutritionally important.

Saccharides are so important that our bodies have developed a backup process for producing the ones in which our diets are deficient. Indeed, using multiple steps, numerous enzymes, and lots of energy-producing molecules such as ATP, most healthy bodies can create every other saccharide from glucose. Enzymes are basically molecular machines that perform energy transfers, converting molecules to new forms—they're in fact the most advanced micromachines ever devised. Xylose, for example, is several steps and enzymes away from glucose. Yet as anyone who has worked in an assembly line knows, it takes just one machine breaking down to shut down the line.

In much the same way, one enzyme not working properly is all that it takes to jam up the works in the body and create inaccurate cell messages. The viruses, bacteria, and environmental toxins that invade our bodies compete for the same vital enzymes that convert saccharides from one form to another. The result, some scientists now believe, is that under stress the body may not be able to manufacture essential saccharides fast enough, creating instead faulty messages by manufacturing inaccurate glycoproteins, the substances that contain sugars and proteins. At first, the body won't work optimally. Eventually, illness may result, particularly if the body is put under unusual or prolonged physical or emotional stress. Supplementing with foods and supplements rich in glyconutrients (see chapter 2) can help prevent potential breakdowns in glycoprotein manufacture and head off illness.

## Multicellular Intelligence

Residing in the brain are as many neurons as stars in the Milky Way. It's estimated that, in total, each of us is made up of 50 to 100 trillion cells, give or take a few trillion. A hundred trillion of anything working together is more complex than any system that human society has ever designed. Scientists have only scratched the surface in understanding how the human body operates and how it keeps its act together. Even the Human Genome Project, the thirteen-year effort by the U.S. Department of Energy and the National Institutes of Health to identify all 100,000 genes in human DNA, is not dealing in trillions of neurons. When thinking about the complexity of the human body, you have to wonder, How do all the cells get along? How do they maintain coherence and cohesion?

The answer lies in communication, and saccharides are an important part of the process. The cells in our bodies use saccharides to communicate with each other—what I call "multicellular intelligence." How important are these sugars? Most people know the four major blood types: O, A, B, and AB. What most people don't realize is that saccharides determine the difference between one blood type and another—and transfusing the wrong blood type can result in illness or death.

From the very beginning of life cells communicate with each other using sugars on the surface of the cell. This complex language is part of the glue that holds the complex system of the human body together—and keeps out what doesn't belong. A woman's egg recognizes suitable healthy sperm of its own species from the complex of saccharides at the tip of the sperm that talk to corresponding sugars and proteins on the surface of the egg cell. A sperm cell from a species different than the egg's will not be welcome: a cat-dog creature will never be created naturally because the cat and the dog eggs and sperm have distinct identities conveyed through saccharides. It is a foolproof insurance against genetic chaos. Saccharides enable cells to give and receive instructions, respond to each other's needs, know when to stop multiplying, and respect each other's space. Virtually every change within our multicellular bodies, from conception until death, is to some degree mediated by this language of sugars.

## Sugars Versus Proteins

Until recently it was thought that pure proteins alone were responsible for cell communication, whereas saccharides were relegated to a lowly status in the nutritional world as cheap and abundant sources of energy. When I was a medical student twenty years ago I was taught that the unusual sugars found on the coats of cells were mostly a nuisance that prevented scientists from studying the precious proteins entombed within them.

We've come a long way in our thinking since then. While there is no doubt that proteins play a cardinal role in cell communication, there are limits to the number of messages they can convey within a limited space. Two identical amino acids, the building blocks of proteins, can combine to form only one biochemical message, whereas two identical monosaccharides can form eleven distinct molecules. But that's only the beginning: Four *different* amino acids can form only twenty-four distinct molecules, whereas four different saccharides can potentially combine into 35,560 distinct molecules called tetrasaccharides.*[24] We now know that each of these 35,560 different tetrasaccharide shapes is potentially a distinct letter in the language of the cells. Saccharides thus have an overwhelming edge in forming molecular messages over the bulkier proteins. They're ideal for transmitting lots of biological information in compact packages, with a distinct advantage over proteins, which require significantly more mass and space to convey the identical amount of biological information.

## Saccharides and Cell Development

Although *no* pregnant or nursing woman should ever take *any* glyconutrient supplements, some laboratory studies on animals indicate that essential saccharides play an important role in fetal cell development and in preventing birth defects. Teratology is the branch of medicine that studies birth defects. It is a word rooted in ancient Greek, from *teras*, meaning "monster." Thus, *teratology* is the study of "monsters," and a *teratogen* is something that creates monstrosities or significant deviations from the norm. Intolerant of those who deviated from the norm, the ancient Greeks sought the perfect human, reflected in their statuary.

---

**Tetra* means "four." Therefore, four monosaccharides joined together form an oligosaccharide called a tetrasaccharide. Five monosaccharides form a pentasaccharide, and so on.

In medical parlance today, a teratogen is any agent that causes birth defects. Teratogens can be genetic or can be caused by chemicals, drugs, radiation, or a shortage of a critical nutrient. Often, the cause of a birth defect in a particular individual is unknown, but one of the most well-documented teratogens is thalidomide. While never approved in the United States, thalidomide was prescribed to pregnant women in England to treat morning sickness and ended up causing stunted or missing limbs in their offspring. It was a textbook teratogen because even one pill could have disastrous consequences.

Exposure to most teratogens, however, does not invariably lead to birth defects. Many babies are exposed; most escape unscathed. For instance, although numerous studies have demonstrated the harmful effects of alcohol on fetal cell development, many women who drink the occasional glass of wine during pregnancy deliver healthy babies. But a minority of babies minimally exposed to alcohol in utero develop fetal alcohol syndrome, in which the newborn exhibits symptoms of alcohol withdrawal and may go on to experience lifelong physical and mental deficits, including short stature, learning disabilities, and hyperactivity. Of course, mothers who drink heavily often give birth to babies who develop this syndrome. Toxic events cause damage to the fetus by interrupting the process of development at crucial junctions during gestation, so obstetricians discourage any alcohol during pregnancy.

What protects an exposed baby from developing fetal alcohol syndrome or problems from other toxic exposures? Why do so many babies skate along, developing normally? What do they have that shields them from harm? We don't know because most medical inquiry focuses on the abnormal event, with the presumption that normal is something that just happens. Another teratogen is folic acid deficiency. Abnormalities in the complete development of the nervous system are more likely in the offspring of mothers deficient in folic acid during pregnancy. Because the body doesn't store folic acid, it's important to consume folic acid daily in food or as a supplement. Clearly, folic acid is crucial in the development of the nervous system, yet the overwhelming majority of babies born to mothers deficient in folic acid during pregnancy are normal. What is protecting these unborn babies? They must have some means to compensate for their inadequate nourishment.

While we don't know how the fetuses manage to thrive, some studies indicate that supplementation with glyconutrients may give the developing embryo an edge when it encounters challenges from teratogens. Two studies on rats point to the possible role of glyconutrients in preventing birth defects and promoting normal development. In 1995, researchers at Shimane Medical University in Japan exposed the entire bodies of pregnant mice to X-rays, a known teratogen, on the seventh day of gestation. Half of the mice were injected with a glyconutrient called polysaccharide K within ten minutes of being irradiated.[25] Since this study was done at the Department of Ophthalmology, the main focus was on fetal eye abnormalities, which tend to be numerous in mice born to X-ray-exposed mothers.

Within seventy-two hours after receiving radiation, the scientists observed that the rat embryos injected with glyconutrients were protected from the early microscopic ocular changes already beginning to occur in the controls. Besides preventing eye defects, the glyconutrients suppressed fetal death, which was common in the controls. Glyconutrients appear to be an equal-opportunity antiteratogen. In another Japanese study, rats were exposed to a chemical called 5-azacytidine (5-AC), which causes finger and toe deformities. Given from twenty-four hours before to one hour after 5-AC treatment, again polysaccharide K significantly suppressed these abnormalities.[26]

## Identity and Intelligence

The most important attribute of a living being is its identity— and saccharides help to preserve it. It's been said that if we reduced a human being to the basic elements that make up the physical body, the whole bucket of stuff—iron, calcium, carbon, water, and the rest—would amount to less than $5 worth of supplies at a hardware store. But constructing a man-made machine with the complexity and capacity of a human being would be prohibitively expensive. The difference between the human being and the hardware-store accoutrements is in the way the human being is put together. Likewise, a pinch of sand and a computer chip are both made of silicon. What makes them different, what gives each a distinct identity, is how they're assembled.

Identity enables us to maintain our uniqueness and complexity in the face of degenerative forces. The body's cells must maintain that identity in stable form for as long as possible to enjoy a long life. Without this stable, physical identity, the body would very quickly dissolve in the face of intrusions from bacteria, viruses, and other organisms. If the boundaries of identity were not being enforced, molecules of saliva from a mosquito bite could invade and confuse your body's cells. Science fiction vividly illustrates extreme forms of identity confusion with stories of disparate DNA commingling in genetic mergings of human and fly to fashion actor Jeff Goldblum's BrundleFly or *Star Trek*'s half-man/half-machine Borg.

## Structure

Our bodies' cells and structures are rebuilt and repaired without cease from conception until death. One drop of blood contains millions of red blood cells; their average life span is 120 days. Every day, blood cells are destroyed and new ones created. A similar process is ongoing in the other tissues of our bodies. We are in a constant process of being rebuilt. Over time, the forces that maintain our structure and identity begin to lose ground to the forces that seek to break us down, and so we age. The secret to a long and healthy life is figuring out how to lay down better, healthier cells than the ones that have passed. One of the lessons emerging from saccharide research is that in some cases we can delay and even reverse the aging process by adding essential saccharides to our diet (see chapter 13).

## Multicellular Intelligence at Work

Forces that predominate on earth tend to push everything to the simplest and most stable form. Oxygen, for example, is a highly reactive element and inherently unstable until it combines with something else in a process called oxidation. Our bodies use that unstable quality of oxygen, its hunger for stability, to generate energy.

But oxygen's unstable quality also generates highly reactive atoms called free radicals that damage our bodies. While we need free radicals to survive—we use them, for instance, to create energy from food—they eventually wear us out. There is a relentless daily struggle between the useful energy-yielding properties of oxidation and its propensity to destroy tissues. Part of our identity intelligence is spent in restraining oxidation within the cell. It is very much like the electricity in your apartment or house. We confine it to insulated wiring that can light our home and power our machines, yet are aware that it can short-circuit and cause damage or even burn down the house. Glyconutrients support the body's ability to neutralize oxidative damage, to insulate the body from damage. Because glyconutrients are not antioxidants like vitamins, however, the function of saccharides is to erect the glycoprotein enzymes that generate the potent antioxidants that keep the body strong.

But they can't do everything. Case in point: In a Japanese study of patients with metastatic cancer (which means that the cancer had spread), one group entered the study well nourished while the other group was poorly nourished. While both groups received glyconutrients as part of their treatment, compared with the well-nourished cancer patients, the poorly nourished patients fared badly.[27] These sugars are not the whole answer; other aspects of nutrition as well as exercise are equally important. In places in the world where there is severe protein deficiency, for instance, adequate saccharide intake on its own is not enough to produce health. The several million new cells that we create every minute of every day need a constant bath of proteins, vitamins, carbohydrates, and hormones. When a cell needs a vital nutrient, it needs it pronto, and if deficiencies persist, generations of new cells will function below par. Glyconutrients are just one piece of the puzzle, one spoke in the wheel toward achieving perfect balance. The body wants to be well; glyconutrients, along with a nutritious diet and exercise, are a vital part of the equation to keep it running smoothly.

## Chapter 2

# The Eight Essential Saccharides

---

*What they do, in what foods and supplements they are found, and what happens if we're deficient.*

In the mid-1980s I was working as a young doctor at a rural Catholic hospital called Shisong, in Cameroon, Africa. One of my senior colleagues was a Swiss doctor named Tony. Multitalented and conscientious, he trained horses and operated on strangulated hernias with equal skill and intensity. One evening Tony invited my family over for dinner, and among the offerings was a dish that included small, wild mushrooms that he had personally picked from the mountain slopes of Switzerland.

Mushrooms can be a great source of nutrition or a potentially deadly poison. As such, they warrant our vigilance and respect. Some species of toadstools, including *Incoybe* and *Clitocybe*, contain a toxin called muscarine, which induces vomiting, cramps, and diarrhea within a few minutes to a few hours after eating. Some patients go on to develop seizures, slip into a coma, and die within a day—although full recovery is possible with swift therapy. Far more dangerous, however, is poisoning caused by the mushroom *Amanita phalloides*, better known by its disquieting nickname the "death cap" mushroom. Within a few hours to a day after consuming the mushroom, the first stage of poisoning begins, characterized by nausea, diarrhea, vomiting, and fever. These overt symptoms subside in stage two, often bringing an evanescent sense of relief to its victims, who may dismiss the problem as an intestinal flu—but all the while their liver and kidney functions steadily deteriorate. In stage three, the liver and or kidney may fail completely; 50 percent of patients die. Although there is no dependable antidote, in some cases organ transplants can be performed.

With all this as a backdrop, my first question to Tony was whether he was knowledgeable about mushrooms. (After all, as the saying goes, there are bold mycologists and there are old mycologists, but there are no old, bold mycologists.) He said yes. Having known Tony for several months, his assurance was good enough for me. I was satisfied that he knew his mushrooms as well as he knew everything else he cared about. I ate the mushrooms with little apprehension.

A couple of months later it was my turn to entertain, and among the dishes I served was mushroom soup made from a local mushroom that grew in the wild, sprouting at the onset of heavy rains. Growing to the size of a medium-size lampshade or a small umbrella, some of those mushrooms weighed 20 pounds or more. In fact, people in the area chopped the mushroom into steak-size pieces and stored them. They made good steaks! Tony asked me what the large chunks of white meat in the soup were. When I replied, "Mushrooms," his eyes widened with worry and his spoon paused halfway to his mouth. "Do you know about mushrooms? Do you know these mushrooms? Are you sure they are edible?" he fired off in rapid succession. (Clearly, in this matter he didn't trust me as much as I had trusted him.) All I could say was that I knew that the local people had been eating these mega-mushrooms for hundreds of years, and they were not getting sick or dying from them. Reluctantly he took my word and ate his soup with the care of someone ingesting Japanese fugu, an exceptionally poisonous saltwater fish that must be prepared by specially trained cooks. (An error in preparation may signify a death sentence, by respiratory paralysis, for those who consume the fish.)

This story came to mind as I thought about how we as humans first came to eat the things that we now do. Imagine our Neolithic ancestors foraging for food. What was it like when they migrated to a new land with unfamiliar plants and animals? They must have been apprehensive as they sampled the plants, animals, edible rocks (yes, edible rocks exist—but that's another story), and insects of the new country, trying to figure out what was edible and what was not. They were not strangers to the thrill that Tony and I felt as we sampled exotic mushrooms. A species that derives pleasure from roller-coasters and bungee jumping surely could not have shrunk from sampling pieces of its environment. Over time, the early people must have determined what caused bellyaches—or worse—and what made them feel good. When they developed agriculture, they narrowed their choices even more, perhaps to those crops that were easiest to cultivate or those that had the greatest yields. In most traditional societies in which people live off the land, there are no pure agriculturists. People retain some aspect of hunting and gathering directly from nature. Tony's knowledge of edible Swiss mushrooms may have been handed down from his ancient mountaineer ancestors.

It follows that all around us are plants and animals that our ancestors used for food but that have been lost to our memory as a race. The variety of flora and fauna on the planet has ensured that there is no standard human food. What we eat today is a result of historical, cultural, and geographical happenstance. It has become nutritional dogma that foods contain vital substances necessary for our survival, including proteins, carbohydrates, fats, vitamins, and minerals. Does that mean that there are no other nutritional categories, that scientists have already identified all that can be known about food and nutrition? On the contrary, we are just beginning to unravel the secrets of how complex and powerful foods really are. Glyconutrients are only now being studied and appreciated. In controlled studies, glyconutrients have been shown to improve healing and immune functioning; help the body fight cancer, viruses, bacteria, and parasites; and improve the functioning of the nervous system without toxic side effects. It's even possible that some of the conditions that we now treat with drugs may actually be manifestations of nutritional deficiencies.

Glyconutrients are raising the bar on what we can expect of human performance and longevity. Two-time NBA most-valuable player Karl Malone takes glyconutrients, as do Olympic basketball star Nancy Lieberman-Cline, Cleveland Indians manager and former ballplayer Mike Hargrove, and gold medal Paralympic sprinter Tony Volpentest, who was born without hands or feet. Glyconutrients took center stage in 1993 at the Chinese National Games, when the nine-member women's running team broke nine world records, one by an astonishing forty-two seconds.[1] Charges of steroid abuse were hurled, but the team passed the drug tests. At a press conference their coach insisted the remarkable results were due to Chinese herbs, the principal ingredient of which was a glyconutrient from the cordyceps mushroom, testimony to the concept that glyconutrients may do more than just help the body to reverse disease or prevent it from occurring in the first place: in some cases, as with the Chinese runners, glyconutrients may increase endurance and vitality beyond our expectations.

As previously stated, glyconutrients are food sources that provide some or all of the eight essential saccharides—mannose, glucose, galactose, fucose, xylose, N-acetylglucosamine, N-acetylgalactosamine, and N-acetylneuraminic acid—necessary for cell-to-cell communication and optimal immune response. Humans have the capability to transform sugars from one form to another, but we can't create sugar on our own. In fact, no animal can: Only plants can create their own sugars, using water, carbon dioxide, and energy from the sun and employing enzymes and energy-trapping chlorophyll in the process known as photosynthesis.

The eight essential saccharides are described in more detail below.

## MANNOSE

I like to compare mannose to a Christmas tree, upon which the other essential saccharides are affixed like ornaments. Mannose is a major player in tissue remodeling and intelligent interactions between cells. The addition of mannose to your diet can accelerate the processes of cellular communication and healing; inhibit tumor growth and spread; and prevent bacterial, viral, parasitic, and fungal infections. It's necessary for the production of cytokines (the chemicals that make us feel achy when we're sick, which the body produces to fight invaders).[2, 3] Research suggests that mannose also eases inflammation in rheumatoid arthritis, and studies on lupus patients indicate a deficiency in this saccharide.[4] Mannose also lowers blood sugar and triglyceride levels in diabetics.[5]

### FUCOSE

Abundant in human breast milk and certain mushrooms, fucose influences brain development. Animal studies using fucose indicate that the saccharide may also help improve the brain's ability to create long-term memories.[6, 7] Fucose is an immune modulator as well, inhibiting tumor growth and its spread and enhancing cellular communication. High concentrations of fucose are found at the junctions between nerves, in the kidney and testes, and in the outer layer of skin.[8] Fucose metabolism is abnormal in cystic fibrosis, diabetes, and cancer and during episodes of shingles, which is caused by a herpes virus. (Shingles is a reactivation of dormant chicken pox virus.) Studies suggest the sugar is active against other herpes viruses, including herpes I and cytomegalovirus. The saccharide also guards against respiratory tract infections and inhibits allergic reactions.[9, 10]

### GALACTOSE

Galactose is abundant in dairy products, where it coexists with glucose in a disaccharide called lactose. In animal studies, galactose inhibits tumor growth and its spread, or metastasis, particularly to the liver.[11] The sugar also enhances wound healing, decreases inflammation, enhances cellular communication, and increases calcium absorption. Galactose supplementation helps protect mice exposed to X-ray radiation from developing cataracts.[12] Galactose levels are usually lower in people with adult and juvenile arthritis and in those with lupus.[13, 14, 15, 16] Studies also indicate that the saccharide triggers long-term memory formation.[17]

## GLUCOSE

Glucose is the ubiquitous saccharide. Table sugar is composed of glucose and another saccharide, fructose. Both saccharides reside in candy bars and cupcakes, ice cream and soft drinks. Bread, rice, pasta, vegetables, cereal, honey, corn syrup, and fruit also supply the sugar. A potent fast-energy source that can be released directly into the bloodstream, glucose also enhances memory, stimulates calcium absorption, and enhances cellular communication. Too much of it can raise insulin levels, leading to obesity and diabetes. Too little glucose can be problematic as well. Elderly Alzheimer's patients, for instance, register much lower glucose levels than those with organic brain disease from stroke or other vascular disease.[18,19, 20, 21] In addition, glucose metabolism is disturbed in depression, manic-depression, anorexia, and bulimia.[22, 23, 24]

## N-ACETYLGALACTOSAMINE

Although research on N-acetylgalactosamine has been limited, we do know that the saccharide inhibits tumor spread and enhances cellular communication. Lower-than-normal levels of this sugar have been found in patients with heart disease.[25]

## N-ACETYLGLUCOSAMINE

N-acetylglucosamine is an immune modulator with antitumor properties and activity against HIV.[26] Glucosamine, a metabolic product of N-acetylglucosamine, helps repair cartilage, decreases pain and inflammation, and increases range of motion in osteoarthritis (see chapter 10).[27, 28] In addition, the saccharide is vital to learning. In one study, researchers found that after two groups of mice received glucosamine injections, the group given fifteen minutes' worth of avoidance-conditioning training (in which they were punished by electric shock for responding to some stimuli and rewarded with food for responding to others) incorporated nearly *double* the amount of glucosamine into their brains as the mice that were not trained and were kept quietly in a cage (see chapter 14).[29] Glucosamine may also help repair the mucosal-lining defensive barrier called the glycosaminoglycan layer, or GAG layer for short. Defects in the GAG layer have been implicated in Crohn's disease, ulcerative colitis, and interstitial cystitis (see chapter 10).[30, 31]

### N-ACETYLNEURAMINIC ACID

Particularly important for brain development and learning, N-acetylneuraminic acid is, not surprisingly, abundant in breast milk. Animal studies indicate that the essential saccharide also improves both memory and performance.[32] In addition, it's an immune modulator that affects the viscosity of mucus, which in turn repels bacteria, viruses, and other pathogens. In several in vitro (Latin for "test tube") and animal studies, the saccharide has been shown to inhibit strains of influenza A and B viruses more effectively than such prescription antivirals as amantadine and ribavirin.[33, 34] It also influences blood coagulation, brain development, and cholesterol levels, lowering LDL, the so-called bad cholesterol. The processing of this sugar is disturbed in Sjögren's syndrome and in alcoholics.[35, 36] In general, levels of this saccharide decrease as we age.

### XYLOSE

An antibacterial and antifungal, xylose also fosters cellular communication. Research suggests that xylose may help prevent cancer of the digestive tract.[37] Xylose absorption is decreased in some patients with intestinal disorders, including colitis.[38, 39] For diabetics and others watching their sugar intake, manufacturers often substitute xylose for sucrose and corn sweeteners in chewing gum and toothpaste. Unlike these sweeteners, xylose does not cause dental cavities.

## Sources of the Eight Essential Saccharides

The health-giving footprints of essential saccharides are found in most folk traditions. In the Western world today, however, of the eight essential saccharides, only glucose and galactose are plentiful in most of our foods. The other six were largely removed from our diets when human beings ceased to be hunters and gatherers and became consumers of a limited variety of processed foods. But they can be found in supplements and some foods—edible fungi, human breast milk, certain fruits and vegetables, unprocessed grains, roots, and plants such as *Aloe vera*. The varied sources of saccharide rich foods and supplements are discussed in detail below.

### ALOE VERA

The medicinal ingredients of the *Aloe vera* plant, a member of the lily family, are contained in the gel within the fleshy leaves. Those ingredients consist of mannose molecules joined together to form a kind of starch or polysaccharide known by a variety of names: acemannan, acetylated polymannans, polymannose, and APM. (For simplicity's sake, we'll call it acemannan.) Health food stores stock topical aloe and *Aloe vera* juice. Aloe is also available in dry powder form, which is used in nutritional supplements.

Aloe's role in accelerating the healing of burns and cuts has been well known for millennia. Potted aloe plants were essential supplies in the campaigns of Alexander the Great. He actually fought a war to procure this prized nutrient to apply to the wounds of his soldiers, capturing an island in the Indian Ocean that's now part of Yemen, called Socotra, which teemed with the plant. Early references to the powers of aloe abound. Verses of the New Testament (John 19:39–40) discuss removing Christ from the cross and wrapping him in a mixture of aloes and myrrh. The Egyptians, including Cleopatra, were among the earliest advocates, as were Hippocrates, King Solomon, Marco Polo, the Aztecs, and the ancient Ayurvedic physicians of India.

These days, the plant is cultivated largely in the Caribbean and southern Africa, and its popularity continues. Recently, a young woman came to my office and proudly showed off a well-healed second-degree burn on her forearm. Her sole treatment, she claimed, consisted of applying the inner gel of fresh *Aloe vera* leaves for a few days, and the aloe, she added, alleviated the pain straightaway.

But aloe has had its share of skeptics, partly because aloe has been hailed as a cure for everything from arthritis and cancer to acne and stretch marks. Some processing techniques extract active substances from the plants with alcohol, yielding a product with none of the medicinal properties of the fresh aloe leaf. The quality of commercial aloe can differ tremendously from bottle to bottle and from producer to producer: if the label doesn't say the aloe is "stabilized," don't buy the product. Without proper processing, a mannose-destroying enzyme is activated every time a leaf is crushed or injured. That enzyme proceeds to digest the polysaccharides on the leaf like a termite digesting wood, and within a day or two, the leaf is useless for healing. We'll explore further the properties of aloe—from wound and burn healing to lowering blood sugar and improving food absorption—later in the book.

### ARABINOGALACTANS

Arabinogalactans, better known as gum sugars, are complex polysaccharides. You can find arabinogalactans in corn, wheat, leeks, carrots, radishes, pears, red wine, coconut meat, and tomatoes, as well as in the medicinal herbs curcumin and echinacea, whose immune stimulatory activity has been linked to its arabinogalactan content.[40] In fact, gum sugars stimulate activity of natural killer cells, interleukins, interferons, and tumor necrosis factor, all key factors in a robust immune response.[41, 42]

The most important single commercial source of the polysaccharide comes from the larch tree. Larch arabinogalactan is an FDA-approved nontoxic food and cosmetics additive. It's also an excellent emulsifier, an agent that uniformly mixes water with fats and oils. Studies indicate that arabinogalactans are particularly effective for digestive problems, as they encourage healthy bacteria in the gut (see chapter 10). They also enhance immune activity and inhibit cancer metastasis to the liver in lymphomas and sarcomas in animal studies (see chapter 11).[43, 44] Gums are also used as food thickeners; they're part of a group of soluble fibers known as mucilages, of which psyllium is also a member. Rich in polysaccharides, psyllium lowers cholesterol[45] (see chapter 15) and is a popular remedy for constipation and irritable bowel syndrome.

## BREAD MOLDS

Bread molds contain small amounts of the saccharide mannose, a minor nutritional source of glyconutrients in the days when bread went moldy routinely and people were often too poor and hungry to worry about moldiness in their food. These days, there are better—not to mention tastier—ways to get glyconutrients.

## BREAST MILK

Human breast milk is rich in glycoproteins and oligosaccharides (which contain three to six monosaccharides). In fact, there are more than 130 different combinations of oligosaccharides in human breast milk. Scientists are beginning to understand just how important breast milk is to immune functioning, from fostering brain development to preventing allergies and infections, including the common rotavirus, which causes diarrhea.[46] Formula-fed infants don't get the quantity and diversity of oligosaccharides present in human breast milk.[47]

## MUSHROOMS

The best-studied glyconutrient mushrooms have been used in the Orient for millennia. In ancient China, Taoist alchemists concocted tonics and teas from these highly regarded foods. The royals and the wealthy were convinced that mushrooms improved health and extended life spans. Indeed, the kidney-shaped reishi—so shiny it looks shellacked—was hailed as the mushroom of immortality. The ancients used it to sharpen memory, improve mood, and enhance vital energy, what the Chinese call *qi*, or *chi.*

Known as ling zhi in China, reishi (its better-known Japanese name) ranges in color from deep red to purple to black; most varieties are bitter, tough, and purely medicinal, not for eating. Not so the fluffy maitake, whose fan-shaped, grayish-brown caps resemble feathers and taste a little like chicken, which is why the mushroom is known by the sobriquet "hen of the woods." In Japan, it's also called the "dancing" mushroom, presumably because those lucky enough to find one—often at the base of a plum, peach, or apricot tree—would be so delighted that they would dance. A maitake mushroom can grow larger than a basketball, though it will weigh considerably more—up to 50 pounds. The earliest written record of its use dates from the Han dynasty in China, from 206 B.C. to A.D. 220, when the fungus was used to treat spleen and stomach problems, hemorrhoids, and anxiety.[48] Later, in feudal times, it was so prized that it was traded for its weight in silver.

These days, most mushrooms are cultivated rather than found. After World War II, the Japanese began drilling holes into logs and packing them with mushroom culture, a process that took eighteen months—too long to be economically practical. Now, many kinds of mushrooms are spawned in sawdust, and the growing time has been cut to a few months. Because mushrooms contain no chlorophyll, they derive all their nutrients from the medium in which they're grown. The cordyceps mushroom, however, doesn't grow naturally on trees and isn't spawned in sawdust. Indigenous to the grassy highlands of Southwest China and Tibet, this club-shaped parasitic fungus survives by infecting an underground moth larva or pupa—though some species of cordyceps prefer insects, truffles, or spiders—where it develops, feeding off and leisurely devouring its host. The pimply, fruity body of the mushroom finally breaks through the caterpillar's head and out to the surface, dispersing its spores.[49]

Rich in glucose, mannose, and galactose polysaccharides, cordyceps is used in China to treat cancer by rousing the immune system to ferret out cancer cells and destroy them (see chapter 11).[50] The well-studied fungus is also used to treat high cholesterol and high blood pressure, lupus, kidney disease, hepatitis, cirrhosis of the liver, asthma, and diabetes—all of which we'll explore in detail. In addition, cordyceps is prized as a tonic by the Chinese to increase athletic performance and sexual desire, claims confirmed in clinical studies (see chapter 13). Chinese cooks mix the delicacy into soups, with the mummified caterpillar and mushroom delicately intertwined.[51]

As natural cordyceps is rare and expensive, cordyceps, like other mushrooms, is now cultured and available in extracts as well. The clinical-sounding Cs-4, known as jinshuibao in China, is a cordyceps extract produced from commercially raised cordyceps fermented in grain broth—without the moth larvae. More than 2,000 people with various illnesses have participated in clinical trials of Cs-4, many of which we'll discuss in upcoming chapters.[52] While the Cs-4 studies point to the saccharide part of the mushroom that prevents and treats disease, other research validates what the ancients already knew: that the whole edible mushrooms, not just the extracts, are protective.[53, 54] As with the extracts, the whole mushroom works by boosting the intelligent activity of the immune system's white blood cells, rather than by directly killing cells.

Other highly regarded and well-studied mushrooms include *Coriolus versicolor*, *Agaricus blazei* (better known as murill), and *Sarcodon*, but they're just a handful of the more than 200 known mushrooms that contain essential saccharides capable of arming the immune system against attack by various pathogens,[55] as we'll explore. Many American supermarkets stock the meaty shiitake mushroom—both fresh and dried are excellent sources of glyconutrients. But unless the mushrooms are very fresh, dried is preferable; as with fresh fruits and vegetables, the nutrients in mushrooms fade as they age. Proper drying helps preserve nutrients. Whether fresh or dried, cook your mushrooms before eating them; otherwise, the glyconutrient molecules tend to stay trapped in the chitin, the "skeleton" of mushrooms, which is akin to the cellulose that forms the fibrous structure of green plants.

Which mushroom is best? The jury's still out, and the potential health-giving properties for most mushrooms have not been clinically tested. It's no wonder: more than 80,000 mushroom species have been identified, yet they represent only an estimated 5 percent of the total species on earth.[56] Common sense dictates that eating a variety of mushrooms and extracts would ensure the best nutrient mix. Adding more mushrooms to your diet is an easy, nutritious way to introduce glyconutrients, though the ubiquitous button mushroom is not a good saccharide source. In fact, several studies have concluded that the mushroom induces benign and cancerous tumors in laboratory animals, particularly if eaten raw.[57, 58] Most extracts and supplements are available online or at better health food stores. Some mushrooms can also be home grown from mail-order kits available online. See the resources section for information on how and where to obtain extracts, supplements, and kits.

### PECTINS

Pectins are another important glyconutrient, derived from fruits such as apples and grapefruit. Rich in the essential saccharide galactose, pectins reduce cholesterol in humans and prostate-cancer metastases in animals, as demonstrated in studies (see chapters 15 and 11, respectively).

## Supplements and Drugs

Second-generation glyconutrients came about when twentieth-century scientists began to see their potential and set about doing what modern scientists do best—extracting and analyzing, looking for the active molecules in ancient cures. Unlike glyconutrients, most drugs that scientists have synthesized have toxic side effects, and there is usually a direct correlation between speed of action and toxicity. (To save a life, speed is sometimes of the essence, so the benefits of a fast-acting, toxic drug may outweigh the risks.) A synthetic compound that works quickly with low toxicity and powerful beneficial effects is rare.

Natural glyconutrients often take more time to work than prescription medications, but they offer significant health benefits without the toxicity. Unless you're allergic to one of the ingredients (1 to 2 percent of people will be allergic to any substance), side effects are few when glyconutrients are taken orally in the recommended doses. For more information, see the Side Effects section in chapter 3.

The following are some of the second-generation glyconutrient agents.

### ACEMANNAN
As we've said, acemannan, a polysaccharide composed mostly of mannose monosaccharides, comes from the *Aloe vera* plant. It's one of the purest glyconutrient polysaccharides, in that it contains no proteins or fat. Pure mannose monosaccharide, however, is poorly absorbed by the human digestive system; in fact, it causes diarrhea. The polysaccharide form, which the body can digest, is abundant in aloe juice, topical gels, and powdered saccharide supplements.

### ACTIVE HEXOSE CORRELATED COMPOUND
Active hexose correlated compound (AHCC) is derived from the shiitake mushroom. Unlike the purer shiitake glyconutrient called lentinan (see "Beta-Glucans," below), AHCC is a relatively crude carbohydrate mix that appears useful in treating liver cancer caused by hepatitis C, a common cause of liver cancer (see chapters 11 and 12).

### BETA-GLUCANS
The cell walls of mushrooms and yeasts, as well as oat, rice, and barley brans, contain polysaccharides in a form known as beta-glucans, which have antitumor, antiviral, antibacterial, antifungal, and antiparasitic actions. In addition, beta-glucans can reduce total cholesterol, triglycerides, and low-density lipoproteins, or LDLs, the so-called bad cholesterol (see chapter 15). In addition to beta-glucans, rice bran contains the polysaccharide arabinoxylane, which has been shown in test-tube studies to increase natural killer cell function.[59] For more on beta-glucans, see "Maitake D-fraction" and "Lentinan."

## BOVINE TRACHEAL CARTILAGE

Although there has been much hoopla over the largely unsupported cancer-curing claims made for shark cartilage, the less-celebrated bovine cartilage from the trachea of cows has shown antitumor efficacy. It is rich in saccharides, and preliminary animal and human studies at Hershey Medical Center at Pennsylvania State University and other universities suggest that it may improve the immune response against many kinds of cancer, including difficult-to-treat ovarian, pancreatic, brain, and kidney malignancies[60, 61] (see chapter 11). And applied topically as an ointment, the glyconutrient has proved effective in accelerating healing after laser skin resurfacing (see chapter 8) to remove wrinkles and acne scars.

None of the three suppliers of bovine tracheal cartilage listed in the resources section use herds from Europe, where mad cow disease has been documented. Lescarden uses cattle from Canada, the United States, and New Zealand. EcoNugenics uses cattle from Australia. And Phoenix Biologics's cattle come from New Zealand and Australia. No cases of people contracting mad cow disease from cattle have been documented in the United States, Canada, New Zealand, or Australia. Cartilage contains no blood vessels or nerve cells, the areas in which mad cow disease is most likely to be concentrated. However, the risk of contracting mad cow disease from bovine tracheal cartilage, while unlikely, has not been scientifically disproved.

## CHITIN AND CHITOSAN

Chitin (pronounced KI·tin) is a polysaccharide composed of the essential sugar N-acetylglucosamine and is found in the shells of crustaceans, including shrimp, krill, and crabs. In the Southern Cameroons, where I was raised, crushed chitin is a popular condiment. Insects, yeast, mushroom cell walls, and certain bacteria cell walls also contain chitin, but these sources haven't been commercialized or studied to the same degree as seafood chitin. Clinical trials indicate that chitin reduces allergic reactions in animals[62] (see chapter 7). Chitosan is chitin modified by acid and alkali. Unlike chitin, chitosan can bind fat and has been found to help people lose weight (see chapter 13). *Do not try chitin or chitosan if you are allergic to shellfish.*

## INULIN AND OLIGOFRUCTOSE

The dahlia plant, chicory, onion, and garlic supply the polysaccharide inulin. Oligofructose is inulin that has been broken down into smaller molecules. Many countries add these fiber-rich glyconutrients to foods to promote colon health. In addition, oligofructose has been shown to reduce the number of colds young children contract in day care (see chapter 5).

## LENTINAN

Lentinan, derived from the cell walls of the shiitake mushroom, is an important beta-glucan. It activates T cells—key players in the immune system that go after tumors, viruses, and other pathogens. Oral lentinan is effective in treating people with venereal warts (see chapter 5). Injectable lentanin has proved helpful in treating chronic fatigue syndrome, cancer, and HIV (see chapters 9, 11, and 12, respectively).

Lentinan administered intramuscularly or intravenously is usually more effective than oral lentinan. Injectable lentinan is available by prescription only and must be administered by a health-care professional. Serious side effects have occured with IV lentinan, and they include fever, chills, back and leg pain, elevated liver enzymes, and anaphylaxis—a serious and potentially fatal allergic reaction.

## LING ZHI-8

Derived from reishi mushrooms, this protein-rich glyconutrient, studies suggest, may have efficacy in treating leukemia. The extract also prevents mice with a predisposition to developing diabetes from getting the disease and has been shown to prevent fatal allergic reactions in rodents—all of which we'll delve into in upcoming chapters. [63, 64]

## MAITAKE D-FRACTION

Maitake D-fraction, a beta-glucan extracted from the maitake mushroom, is exceptionally potent. Researchers have discovered that when given by injection or orally it ameliorates the side effects of chemotherapy, including nausea, vomiting, diarrhea, hair loss, pain, and low white-cell count (see chapter 11). In addition, studies indicate that the compound inhibits cancer and its spread.[65, 66]

## POLYSACCHARIDE K AND POLYSACCHARIDE P

Both polysaccharide K and polysaccharide P are extracted from the *Coriolus versicolor* mushroom, which grows in the wild on tree trunks in North America and Asia. Known in Japan as kawaratake, which translates to "mushroom by the river," and in China as yun zhi or "cloud fungus," *Coriolus versicolor,* commonly known as the turkey-tail mushroom, is woody and fibrous; it's used in teas and extracts, rather than for eating.

Polysaccharide K is also called PSK and krestin; it has been studied extensively since the 1960s in Japan where it is approved to treat cancer. The glyconutrient is often used there in conjunction with traditional cancer treatment, as it has been found to work synergistically with chemotherapy and radiation. Polysaccharide K is slowly gaining popularity in the United States. Polysaccharide P, also known as PSP, was first isolated from the *Coriolus versicolor* mushroom in China, where it is used to treat cancer. It has many of the same properties as its close cousin polysaccharide K. For more information, see chapter 11.

# The Third Generation of Glyconutrients— Saccharide Complexes

These complexes are polysaccharide dietary supplements that contain most or all of the eight essential saccharides. They're obtained from various sources, including rice, barley, and oat brans; mushrooms; yeast cell walls; *Aloe vera*; and gum sugars. The more essential saccharides you add to your diet, the fewer number of steps, enzymes, and energy the body expends processing them for use. As discussed in chapter 1, most healthy people can generate every other essential saccharide from glucose. But if the person is sick or stressed, the body may not be able to marshal the resources it needs to convert one sugar to another. Supplying all eight essential saccharides takes the burden off an overstressed body.

## The Future: Gene Therapy and Nutritional Tailoring

Each of us is equipped with some 30,000 genes. The expression of these genes is what makes us who we are. They give us individuality. They give us identity. Different combinations and types of food are appropriate for different individuals. The foods that are good for us change over a lifetime and during particular periods of our lives. Foods that are not genetically appropriate are likely to affect your health adversely. The expression "One man's meat is another man's poison" is true in some cases.

Some researchers believe that saccharide supplementation may increase expression of important genes thought to be dormant. In the future, glyconutrient research is likely to discover individual saccharide blends finely tailored to complement each person's particular genetics, diet, and lifestyle. In the meantime, however, we know enough about the health-giving aspects of glyconutrients to add them to your diet safely and effectively.

**Chapter 3**

# Nutritional Supplements

---

*The case for them—and against*

Like many physicians, I used to be unreceptive to the idea of nutritional supplementation. And while I believe they have helped me tremendously, there are pros and cons to taking supplements and good reasons for us all to be skeptical and careful.

## The Case Against Supplementation

One of the most powerful arguments against taking vitamins and supplements is that they are naturally available in a good diet. Because an excess of what the body needs of water-soluble vitamins is excreted, supplementation results in "expensive urine." Studies indicate that manufactured vitamins don't provide the same spectrum of benefits or provide the same protection as naturally occurring vitamins in foods.

Recently, the findings of the Framingham Study—long-term

research begun in the late 1960s to assess the effects of fruits and vegetables on stroke risk—demonstrated that while a diet low in both beta-carotene and vitamin C nearly doubles the risk for stroke, chugging down vitamins is not the solution. Quite the contrary—strokes were *more* frequent in the group that used vitamins than in those who did not. The solution, according to this study, is a diet rich in fruits and vegetables. People who consumed three or more servings of fruits and vegetables daily had a 22 percent lower risk of stroke and were half as likely to die from a stroke, should one occur. In addition to failing to provide the nutrients found in food, many supplements aren't well absorbed or assimilated and are of doubtful efficacy.

Another argument against supplement use is that many of the formulations on the market have no clinical studies to support their claims. Some manufacturers tend to mix compounds into a tablet without testing their efficacy.

Finally, in Western culture, the word *vitamin* has come to connote an almost mythical power. Hope springs eternal that undiscovered nutritional substances in nature will prolong life indefinitely. But nothing is better than getting your nutrients through your food. Sometimes, however, if natural, organic, nutrient-rich foods are not available, supplements are necessary.

## The Case for Supplementation

Compared with the diets of our Neolithic hunter-gatherer ancestors, what we eat today is limited and usually highly processed. The foods that made their way into agricultural practice are largely the result of historical accident, commercial interest, convenience, agricultural know-how, and cultural selection. How many Americans would indulge in grasshoppers, locusts, or crickets— nutritious delicacies in various other parts of the world? Yet without childhood conditioning and slick marketing, most people wouldn't touch hamburgers or hot dogs, either.

As new nutrients are discovered, Western consumers generally add supplements to their usual diets rather than increase their servings of fruits and vegetables. Also, genetic variety is actively being bred out of our current agricultural stocks. With fewer choices we are likely to get fewer of the nutrients that we need. The cultivation of different strains of crops is based on market demand, which is determined not so much by nutritional value as by taste, shelf life, and productivity.

Cultural bias, ingrained habits, and our restless, mobile life-style and lack of time to prepare healthy meals make it likely that many people will continue to consume overprocessed foods that are low in nutritional value. Even in our overfed Western society there is a pervasive undernutrition. Many people caught in this cycle of less-than-optimal nutrition will swallow a nutritional supplement rather than adopt foods that they don't like or that require self-discipline, cooking time, or expertise to prepare.

Ill health stems not only from what's in the junk food we eat but also from what's missing. Nutritional supplementation can help fill the gaps in our nutrition. It's not a perfect system, but for most of us mortals lapses in good nutrition are a given. Developing better nutritional supplements is a compromise alternative. By this I don't mean to suggest that being poorly nourished is okay as long as you take supplements—no supplement can do much good if your diet is bad. The chain of practices that affects your health is only as strong as its weakest link.

Another reason to take supplements is that they're getting better. Nutraceuticals are nutritional supplements that have proven health benefits. Organizations such as the American Nutraceutical Association, which publishes the latest science on these supplements, are influencing the standardization of supplements and ensuring the constancy of their composition. New high-tech methods can extract micronutrients without the denaturing that weakens or destroys their nutritional value. It seems reasonable that someone who can't stomach salads should be able to consume a tablet or a powder that contains the nutrients and benefits of fruits and vegetables—provided that the tablet or powder does indeed contain what its packaging says it does.

Besides, there's a Luddite feeling in the concept that we can get all we need from a certain kind of balanced diet. It denies the inquiring spirit that has brought us medical advances such as antibiotics, which have saved millions of lives, and research, which has led to heart transplants and other life-saving treatments. The fact is that nature did not hand over to humanity everything that we've needed in our diets. We had to develop agriculture to make food supplies more predictable and less subject to the vagaries of climate and weather, which can still challenge our ability to reap enough of a harvest. Our ancestors deliberately selected grains that could be stored and meats that could be dried and preserved, rather than highly perishable foods, for their diets.

In the past seventy-five years researchers have devised a host of refinements in food manufacturing that increase shelf life, improve taste, and make food widely available. By processing foods, however, we deplete nutrients and then add unnecessary sweeteners and artificial flavors. In commercial cereals, vitamins that processing has eliminated are often added back in. This kind of manipulation is just at its infancy, compared with what will be the norm twenty years from now, when genes added to plant varieties and animal stocks will attempt to confer additional nutritional benefits to foods. There is nothing "natural" about most of the foods we eat. Much of the diet we eat and prefer today is the result of a combination of agricultural development and selection, history, geography, the intersection of cultural tastes—and marketing.

Because of all these trends and factors, nutritional deficiencies, mostly unrecognized, are embedded within our current dietary mix. Our Western diet, for instance, is deficient in vitamin E. Our current choices of foods in America have significantly evolved beyond what people ate as recently as the 1950s.

## Gong

*Gong* is a Chinese term that means cultivation, as in personal cultivation. It also connotes perfect balance, holistic harmony. And kung-fu or gong-fu is a practice in which martial arts proficiency is built up by practicing a set of skills daily in a focused and nonobsessed manner. A little practice daily with incremental addition of range, speed, and techniques without strain is the aim of any gong. Through daily practice one builds on the previous day's gains without getting hurt.

Good nutrition, like kung-fu, must be practiced every day to get the benefits, unlike taking medication, which requires a fixed dose and usually a limited course of treatment. Supplements may be part of the gong. In the past, nutritional science worked backward from states of nutritional deficiency to find out what was minimally necessary to prevent those deficiencies. Yet today science is exploring the possibility that we can go beyond being just okay to functioning at our very best and perhaps even beyond what were previously accepted as our limits. Nutritional science is looking for ways to convey optimal health.

Traditional healers, particularly those of traditional Chinese medicine, used good nutrition and supplements in pursuit of healing and optimum wellness. This ancient system asked: How do we maintain a high state of health for as long as possible? How do we defeat disease and aging by using nutrition, exercise, and meditation? What are our true limits of human mortality? How can we reach them? How can we exceed them?

Modern science is giving us the tools to answer these questions but needs to remember to work with the traditional medical philosophies that recognize the innate self-healing tendency of the human cells. The body wants to be well; a body in tip-top condition uses less energy and is more efficient. Homeostasis—the drive toward equilibrium, balance, and harmony—is built into living systems.

In his book *The Book of Ginseng and Other Herbs for Vitality*, Dr. Stephen Fulder writes, "The ancient medical system built upon the Taoist view of health taught that the primary activity should be to establish harmony so as to avoid disease."[1] The ancient sages did not focus on those who were sick, but rather on those who were well, in order to learn how to keep them that way.

In fact, doctors were enjoined to maintain the health of their patients before anything else. This was what they were paid for. If the patient fell ill, it was deemed to be partly the doctor's fault. Payments would cease, and the doctor was considered ignorant.[2] (I wonder what would happen if we reversed the Western system and began paying doctors only when we were healthy?) The inferior physician, according to *The Yellow Emperor's Classic of Internal Medicine*, a book on the art of healing written sometime between 221 and 206 B.C., begins to help when destruction has already begun.

Natural supplements work with the body's self-healing functions to get the body back to homeostasis. With supplements, Western medical technology works together with Eastern healing philosophy to maintain wellness and help the body to heal.

In today's world, we face an entirely different set of health challenges from those of even fifty years ago. New toxins in our environment and food called xenosubstrates, which our bodies were not designed to handle, compete with normal substrates—the food or other ingested substances in the body—for valuable enzymes, which are usually proteins or glycoproteins. Enzymes convert substrates into a form desired by the body to achieve a certain end, such as nourishment, tissue repair, or energy. When xenosubstrates use up precious enzymes, our bodies try to meet the challenge by upregulating, producing more enzymes to offset the effects of the toxins. Creating more enzymes depends on the presence of appropriate raw materials, including saccharides.

In a world devoid of toxins, drugs, and other xenosubstrates, the body's innate process for obtaining additional saccharides would in most cases suffice. In today's world, confronted as we are by levels and varieties of chemicals never before encountered by human biochemistry, the need for saccharides may not always be satisfied by the backup process alone and supplements may be needed to fill in the gaps. For instance, as discussed in chapter 1, when pregnant rats were exposed to a toxic chemical—a prime example of a xenosubstrate—and then given glyconutrients, they were less likely to develop birth defects.[3] Similarly, pregnant mice exposed to radiation, but protected by glyconutrients, are less likely to produce offspring with birth defects.[4]

While glyconutrient studies on animals and people have been

impressive, many glyconutrients have yet to be studied for their specific healing properties. That doesn't mean other glyconutrients won't work as well—or better—for a particular illness than the ones that have been studied, but since they haven't been tested, we don't know for sure.

## The Dos and Don'ts of Taking Glyconutrients

Consult your health-care provider before adding glyconutrients to your diet, especially if you have health problems, are prone to allergies, or are taking any medications. Pregnant women and women who are nursing should *never* take glyconutrients without consulting their doctor. Glyconutrients can lower blood pressure and blood sugar, so if you're on medications to control either, always consult your doctor before trying glyconutrients. Read labels carefully when purchasing glyconutrients. To enhance flavor, some manufacturers add sweetener, which diabetics and those watching their weight should avoid.

### SIDE EFFECTS

For some people, loose bowel movements or soft stools are normal when using glyconutrients, particularly when first beginning. Mild cramping and gas, which usually subside within a few days to a few weeks, are also normal side effects for some people. If you experience these effects, cut back on your intake or take the glyconutrients only with meals. Some research suggests that supplementing with vitamin C (500 milligrams once or twice daily) will curtail these digestive problems. Very occasionally, polysaccharide K causes a benign darkening of the fingernails.

Allergic reactions to glyconutrient supplements and foods that supply glyconutrients occasionally occur, so pay attention to your body as you take them. In fact, you should pay attention to your body's reactions whenever you try a new food or supplement. From 1 to 2 percent of the population is allergic to any given substance. If you are allergic to any of the ingredients listed on the glyconutrient label, do not take the product. If you are allergic to shellfish, do *not* try chitin or chitosan, as both are made from shellfish. Some allergies, of course, are unforeseen, which makes it important for you to start out slowly. Allergy symptoms for any substance range from the mild to the life-threatening and include hives, rash, shortness of breath, and wheezing. If you experience any of these symptoms while taking glyconutrients, stop taking them and consult your doctor immediately.

In the course of this book, I suggest glyconutrient intakes for particular illnesses—but the amounts I suggest are averages. At a recent Johns Hopkins nutrition conference that I attended, health-care professionals discussed obtaining good results with amounts higher than these averages for some oral glyconutrients. Even so, I have based my recommendations on the many human clinical studies and case reports that I have read, many of which are cited in *Sugars That Heal.*

The medical and scientific communities are still in the early stages of figuring out glyconutrient ranges; there seems to be a lot of leeway, and much individuality. Some people, including those who are more muscular, physically very active, or have a chronic illness, may need more glyconutrients than the average. In particular, some patients with cancer, advanced HIV disease, severe hepatitis, or cirrhosis may require higher-than-average amounts, but this should be determined with a physician's help. If, however, you are sensitive to drugs and foods, are small or thin, or don't exercise, you may need less than the average.

Please take glyconutrients only with your own physician's knowledge and consent if you are under a doctor's care. Whatever dose you and your doctor believe is right for you, *build up gradually over a period of a few weeks.* If you are combining two glyconutrients, cut the dose for each by half; if you combine three glyconutrients, cut the dose for each by two-thirds, and so on. Slow and steady wins the race.

If you are allergic to mushrooms, do not use them as your source for glyconutrients. In addition, several kinds of mushrooms, including cordyceps and reishi, contain the nucleotide adenosine. A structural unit of our DNA, adenosine thins the blood. Pectins have blood-thinning effects as well. Do not take pectins, mushrooms, or their extracts if you have a bleeding disorder or are on a blood thinner, including Coumadin, heparin, or Plavix or if you're taking a Cox-2 inhibitor (Vioxx, Celebrex, or Mobic) unless your doctor gives you the go-ahead, because excessive thinning of the blood can lead to hemorrhage. If you are taking aspirin or prescription or over-the-counter nonsteroidal anti-inflammatory drugs (NSAIDs) such as ibuprofen, Motrin, Aleve, or Naprosyn, consult with your doctor before trying pectins, mushrooms, or mushroom extracts as well. Your doctor may need to adjust your drug dose if you want to try glyconutrients or you may have to turn to other good sources for glyconutrients, including rice, oat, or barley beta-glucans, gum sugars, and *Aloe vera.*

Do *not* take glyconutrient supplements if you are taking the prescription anti-inflammatory indomethacin (Indocin). A recent Japanese study found that injected yeast beta-glucans in combination with an oral dose of indomethacin caused fatalities in mice.

Throughout the book, the recommended intakes listed are for adults, unless otherwise specified. Do not administer glyconutrients to children under twelve without consulting your physician. Children two and under should be administered glyconutrients *only* under the supervision of a physician, because glyconutrients can cause allergic reactions. For children two and above, the dose is *half* the manufacturer's *lowest recommended dose* for adults. Children should *not* take therapeutic amounts of any glyconutrient. In addition, children should not take polysaccharide K, polysaccharide P, and injectable lentinan, as these glyconutrients have not been adequately tested in children, and toxic effects with injectable lentinan have been reported.

To improve your overall health, variety in your diet is beneficial. Include several glyconutrient-rich foods, including mushrooms, garlic, onions, corn, wheat, leeks, carrots, radishes, pears, coconut meat, tomatoes, beans, figs, peas, and slow-cooked oatmeal in your diet, rather than just one or two such foods. Or supplement your favorite mushrooms with a saccharide formula. (See the resources section for available preparations.)

Glyconutrients, like many natural medicines and some prescription drugs, take time to work. While most people experience improvement within a month to six weeks, in some cases it may take up to three months before you experience the full benefits. Some people, however, respond quickly to glyconutrients—within a week or two.

Whenever possible, buy organic mushrooms. Mushrooms tend to concentrate heavy metals, including lead, if these substances are present in the growth medium. It is better to purchase dried mushrooms than fresh unless you eat them within a week of purchase. Drying does not degrade the glyconutrient content of the mushroom; in fact, it preserves the nutrients. Raw mushrooms convey fewer benefits than cooked because the glyconutrient molecules tend to stay trapped in chitin, the polysaccharide that forms the skeleton of mushrooms. So, sauté, bake, stir-fry, grill, or broil your mushrooms. The most certain way to extract the polysaccharides is to prepare a mushroom decoction (tea): Place mushrooms in a pot and add water to cover. Bring to gentle boil. Reduce to a simmer, cover, and cook until the mushrooms are tender. Drink the broth and eat the mushrooms.

Extracts from mushrooms and brans are concentrated, so you need less. For instance, the average intake of maitake extract is 1 to 3 grams (1 gram equals 1,000 milligrams) per day for healthy people, and 3 to 6 grams for those with an acute or chronic disease. But if you choose fresh maitake mushrooms (or powdered maitake mushrooms), you may find you can eat up to a quarter-pound to a half-pound of mushrooms a day. Two hundred grams is 0.44 of a pound, a little less than a half-pound.

Glyconutrients—especially fresh or dried mushrooms and their extracts—can be expensive. For instance, a bottle of sixty 500-milligram capsules of concentrated maitake extract will run about $25. Some mushroom suppliers offer dried mushrooms and mushroom powder in bulk (see the resources section), which is less expensive. More affordable, first-rate sources of glyconutrients include pectins, psyllium, yeast beta-glucans, and rice, oat, and barley brans.

So here you have some of the arguments on both sides of the nutritional supplement issue. If you decide that supplements aren't for you, consider adding more glyconutrient-rich food to your diet by eating more rice, barley and oat brans and mushrooms such as shiitake, maitake, and oyster.

# PART II

# STRENGTHEN YOUR IMMUNE SYSTEM

"It's a pity to shoot the pianist when the piano is out of tune."

—*Rene Coty, President of France, 1953–1959*

## Chapter 4

# Introduction to
# the Immune System

*A brief compendium of the overactive, the underactive, and
the confused.*

**H**uman and animal studies indicate that glyconutrients help the
immune system whether it is overactive—as in lupus, rheumatoid
arthritis, ulcerative colitis, and other autoimmune illnesses—or
underactive, cancer and AIDS being primary examples. That's
why glyconutrients have been called immunomodulators; immunomodulators downregulate the immune system when it is
too active and upregulate when the immune system is not pulling its weight. But I think the term *immunomodulator* is not quite
right because it assumes that the saccharides on their own have
the intelligence to immunomodulate. What saccharides do is to
cause the DNA and the cells themselves to immunomodulate.
Once again, you can see the homeostatic effect of these nutrients.

When empowered, the immune system can more readily identify and destroy what doesn't belong in the body, reinforcing the
body's identity and restoring health. When the immune system fails to perform these functions efficiently, it is, in a word,

dysfunctional. If the immune system seems to be doing nothing while viruses, bacteria, and cancers run rampant, the dysfunction is called an immunodeficiency.

Cancer and AIDS are immunodeficiencies, and chronic fatigue syndrome, Gulf War syndrome, and fibromyalgia appear to be immunodeficiencies as well, though some patients also exhibit symptoms of a disordered immune system, the hallmark of autoimmune diseases. With autoimmunity—the opposite of immunodeficiency—the body seems to be under attack from itself. Usually the phenomenon is characterized as an overactive immune system, but I prefer to think of it as a confused immune system. Why the immune system becomes disordered isn't clear. Various toxins, from mercury to dioxin to insecticides like chlordane, have been implicated, as have vaccines and a host of viral, bacterial, and parasitic agents.

Saccharides are often effective at treating diseases caused by both underactive and confused immune systems because saccharides influence communication between white blood cells and the chemicals they produce. The workings of white blood cells, which compose the immune system, are complicated and interconnected, but don't be concerned if you have trouble grasping the details. It's the fundamental protective actions of the immune system that are important.

## Neutrophils

Small, mobile, and abundant, neutrophils are the first immune cells to arrive on the scene, moving in quickly and in large numbers, gobbling up bacteria and dead tissue. Like kamikaze pilots, neutrophils attempt to destroy their foe—and die in the process. The downside to neutrophils is that they're relatively unsophisticated, so invading organisms with stealth capability can elude them. Still, they're the most abundant immune cells in the blood—they're phagocytes, or eating cells. When they die, they release an enzyme that dissolves cells in the immediate area, resulting in pus formation. That's why they're also called pus cells; pus, which consists of dead cells, is the end result of their efforts.

When they're functioning properly, neutrophils arrive within thirty minutes of an injury, programmed to consume a large array of invaders, thereby reducing the mass of intruders with which the other guardians of the immune system, including the macrophages, would otherwise have to contend. Glyconutrients increase the magnitude and speed with which neutrophils are mobilized, as well as their effectiveness.[1]

## Macrophages

Macrophages are the largest white blood cells in the body, and their main business is to analyze and ingest pathogens. In the liver, for example, macrophages constitute up to 10 percent of the weight of the organ and serve as a formidable trap for microbes. Activated in the immune response, they act as messengers and triggers to coordinate body defense, healing, growth, and remodeling—and glyconutrients influence their production.[2]

Scientists used to think that eating pathogens was the only function of macrophages. Now we know that they perform vital regulatory functions. The macrophage becomes specialized in the affairs of the tissue that it patrols, checking on the health of its cells. It performs that function by "reading" the Braille of the cells' surface, feeling around on the glycoprotein cell coating, checking if the cells are healthy, infected, damaged, or cancerous. Unlike the short-lived neutrophils, the macrophages are relentless and long-lived, capable of such Herculean feats as clutching large foreign objects for months while endeavoring to digest them. Macrophages in the lung, for example, will cleave to the bacteria that cause tuberculosis for months or even years, trying to break them down and preventing them from moving around freely.

Macrophages are the block captains of your neighborhood watch society, the *chefs de quartier* in French-speaking cities.

Monitoring for trouble, sanitation, services, and the general interest of their constituents, they sometimes enlist help from other cells to solve community problems.

Glyconutrients boost the rate, speed, magnitude, and precision of macrophage function, revving up their ability to identify and destroy tumor cells, bacteria, fungi, parasites, and viruses, including those that cause HIV, measles, influenza, and the common cold. Exposure to glyconutrients per se does not cause macrophages to go wild, eating everything in sight. But when there is reason to act, macrophages do so more quickly and vigorously, with more killing power. Macrophages incubated in extracts from the reishi mushroom, for instance, normalize leukemic cells and restore their functions.[3] Other glyconutrients, including maitake D-fraction, acemannan, and arabinogalactans, enhance macrophage activity as well.[4, 5] But free radicals, generated when the macrophages do their work, can reduce the effectiveness of the macrophage and shorten its life span. Macrophages are able to recover from free-radical damage—if they can generate the antioxidants necessary to eliminate them. And again that's where saccharides come in: polysaccharide K, reishi mushrooms, and acemannan, among other glyconutrients, have been shown to increase the enzyme glutathione synthetase, which in turn produces the powerful antioxidant, glutathione.[6, 7, 8]

## Natural Killer Cells

Like vampires, cancer cells and virus-infected cells attain a parasitic immortality at the expense of the rest of the body—and natural killer cells are their enemies, the vampire slayers, with the keen intelligence to detect them. Unlike the macrophage, the natural killer cell does not ingest microbes; it just kills them by dissolving the target cell's cytoplasm with enzymes. Along with macrophages, natural killer cells traverse the tissues to ensure their health. It is part of the redundancy of the human body to ensure that no threat to its identity is missed. The body tends to overdo vital functions, going after the same effect from a slightly different angle, in case one approach fails.

Natural killer cells malfunction in many illnesses, including AIDS, cancer, and chronic fatigue syndrome, with reduced killing power and an accelerated form of programmed cell death.[9, 10] That's the bad news. The good news is that the number and activity of natural killer cells increase significantly when exposed to glyconutrients. In particular, cordyceps, rice bran, and maitake mushrooms have been shown to increase natural killer cell production and effectiveness.[11, 12, 13]

## T and B Cells

While the macrophages, neutrophils, and natural killer cells are army grunts programmed to respond to a wide array of dangers instantly, the lymphocytes, better known as T and B cells, are well-trained specialists. B cells head up the body's *humoral immunity*: these cells produce the antibodies that float in the blood and neutralize or destroy unwanted particles or organisms. T cells are in charge of *cellular immunity*: they are the immune cells that personally take charge of neutralizing a challenge by identifying and killing it. Helper T cells stimulate an immune response, whereas suppressor T cells stop it after the infection has been eradicated. In autoimmune diseases there are usually too many helper cells and not enough suppressor cells, whereas in immunodeficiency diseases like cancer and AIDS, suppressors far outnumber helpers. Glyconutrients help restore the proper balance.

In a Vanderbilt University study, when cells called killer or cytotoxic T cells were fed glyconutrients, both their number and their capacity to destroy a challenge increased dramatically.[14] T cells can't recognize invaders without help from macrophages or monocytes—white blood cells that circulate in the bloodstream for twenty-four hours, after which time they settle into tissues and become macrophages. When T cells are placed in proximity to monocytes that have been exposed to glyconutrients, they become very efficient.[15] Glyconutrients also increase antibody production by B cells.

## Cytokines and Glyconutrients

*Interleukins, tumor necrosis factor, lymphokines,* and *interferons* are all cytokines, the proteins that make us feel achy when we're sick as they combat pathogens. Produced in minute quantities by various cells in the body, they convey messages that cause certain cells to become hypervigilant at spotting invaders. For instance, interferons, which are used to treat hepatitis, multiple sclerosis, Kaposi's sarcoma, and venereal warts, enable T cells to recognize and kill infected cells more easily. Glyconutrients enable our cells to generate more cytokines.[16] When glyconutrients are added to macrophages, for example, the result is increased production of tumor necrosis factor, among other cytokines.[17] Abbreviated TNF, tumor necrosis factor gets its protracted name from its capacity to shut down a tumor's blood supply, resulting in tumor death, or necrosis. The interleukin cytokines cause some cells to proliferate and others to be suppressed and have been used experimentally to treat cancer. Glyconutrients are effective at stimulating interleukin production as well.[18, 19]

Glyconutrients help the immune system function, bestowing beneficial effects on the performances of key immune-system components, from the macrophages, neutrophils, and natural killer cells to antibody and cytokine production. An immune system that's humming along taking care of business, killing the bad guys and watching over the good, helps keep the body healthy in both the short and long term.

## Chapter 5

# Preventing the Common Cold and Other Viruses

*From colds to influenza, condyloma to herpes I and II, glyconutrients help fight viruses.*

**A** virus is the ultimate parasite. It is a tiny life form that cannot perform the majority of life functions on its own. It cannot reproduce; it cannot generate energy; it cannot feed or survive without using the living cell of a higher life form. Most cellular life forms can be infected by some kind of virus. There are viruses that specialize in hijacking bacteria; other viruses prefer plant cells, and still others fancy humans and other animals. Some viruses, like chicken pox and measles, always elicit large, efficient immune responses from the body. Other viruses, including Ebola, smallpox, and yellow fever, cause virulent illness before the body can mount an effective response. Long-lived herpes viruses cause chronic or recurrent disease. Over time, by inserting genes called oncogenes in their host, herpes viruses can cause cells to become cancerous. Influenza and HIV change their composition like chameleons change color; the immune system has a hard time keeping up.

# Colds

## OLIGOFRUCTOSE

Although it causes mischief and misery, the virus that causes the common cold does not kill. Unlike the viruses that cause HIV or hepatitis B or C, which can be transmitted only through contact with blood, saliva, or other bodily fluids, a rhinovirus (the scientific term for the cold virus) is far easier to catch, and can be transmitted with a handshake, a cough, or a sneeze. It's an elusive virus that has no cure. You just have to let it run its course.

The cold virus exists in numerous genetic strains. While you do develop immunity to many strains, there are always many more against which you have no antibodies. That is why we keep catching colds all our lives. (Like other viruses, they're are not affected by antibiotics.) For researchers to develop a vaccine against the common cold they'd have to make it to fight dozens of different strains at once. Imagine all of the suffering—not to mention the loss of productivity at work and the loss of money spent on cold-relief products—that could be avoided if colds could be prevented.

Like other viruses, the human rhinovirus infects by first attaching to specific receptors on the surfaces of its host cells. Glyconutrient research from the late 1980s suggested that wheat-germ lectin, protein molecules that bind or attract saccharides, could prevent a rhinovirus from attaching itself to receptors, thus thwarting a cold.[1] Now, Johns Hopkins studies published in 1999 confirm the ability of saccharides to prevent colds in children.[2, 3] Inulin is a polysaccharide derived primarily from the dahlia plant, chicory, onion, and garlic. Oligofructose is inulin that has been broken down into smaller molecules. (Many countries—though not the United States, as yet—use both inulin and oligofructose to add dietary fiber to foods and to promote colon health.) In one of the Johns Hopkins studies, researchers evaluated oligofructose's effects on 140 babies and toddlers, ages four months to two years, who were in day care and thus at higher risk for contracting illnesses. Specifically, the researchers were investigating whether such gastrointestinal problems as diarrhea, colic, and gas increased or decreased with oligofructose supplementation.

One group of children had oligofructose added to their cereal; the other group received placebo. On average, each child received 1.1 gram of the nutrient daily; dosages were calibrated according to age and weight. The scientists discovered no difference in diarrheal illnesses in both groups, except that the children on oligofructose had significantly fewer episodes of fever accompanying the diarrhea. And there was no difference in vomiting, flatulence, or how many stools they passed every day.

However, what the scientists weren't expecting to find was that the children on oligofructose had far fewer colds than those on placebo. And when the children taking glyconutrients did contract colds, they had fewer instances of fever, required fewer antibiotics for secondary infections, and had fewer doctor visits. These differences were statistically significant, which means there was no doubt that oligofructose had a powerful effect in increasing the body's resistance to colds and in reducing the severity of the cold when one occurred. (See Table 1, below.) While oligofructose is considered safe, one case of an anaphylactic reaction, a serious and potentially fatal allergic reaction, has been described in the literature.

| TABLE 1. INCIDENCE AND EFFECTS OF COLDS IN CHILDREN GIVEN OLIGOFRUCTOSE VERSUS PLACEBO | Oligofructose | Placebo |
|---|---|---|
| Fever and cold symptoms (average number of episodes per child per year) | 11.4 | 17.16 |
| Runny nose (average number of episodes per child per year) | 38.9 | 42.0 |

|                                                                    | Oligofructose | Placebo |
|--------------------------------------------------------------------|:-------------:|:-------:|
| Antibiotic use<br>(average number of episodes per<br>child per year) |     8.24      |  12.18  |
| Day-care absenteeism<br>(average number of days absent<br>per child per week) |     0.31      |  0.79   |

*Suggested Use:* Oligofructose is available only to commercial vendors, but inulin is available to consumers. (See the resources chapter for more information.) The *adult* maintenance dose of inulin for preventing colds and boosting the immune system is 500 milligrams to 1,500 milligrams in divided doses with water. Adults can double their intake if they feel a cold coming on. Adding garlic or onion to your foods and chicory to your coffee will supply inulin naturally. Mild gastrointestinal discomfort, including gas, cramping, and diarrhea are possible side effects with inulin, as with all glyconutrients, particularly when you first begin. If you experience these symptoms, cut back on your intake or take with meals. Some evidence suggests that taking 500 milligrams of vitamin C once or twice daily along with your glyconutrients will curtail these digestive problems.

Always consult with your doctor before administering glyconutrients—including inulin—to children. Glyconutrients should not be administered to children under age two unless under a doctor's supervision. The child's dose for inulin that you can ask your doctor about is 250 milligrams to 500 milligrams daily, in equally divided doses. This dose is *half* the manufacturer's recommended dose for adults. Children should never be given injectable glyconutrients such as lentinan, nor should they take polysaccharide K or P. For more information, see chapter 3.

## RECURRENT COLDS: A PATIENT'S SUCCESS

When Sondra brought her three-year-old daughter, Haley, in to see me because of yet another bad cold, I could see that Haley was out of sorts and Sondra was frustrated. This cold, like many of the rest, was characterized by congestion, cough, and fever. On top of the cold, Haley had developed a secondary bacterial ear infection for which she needed antibiotics. No doubt one of the reasons Haley was plagued with colds—five in eight months— was that her mother runs a day care at home, the perfect breeding ground for viruses and bacteria.

Sondra wanted to know if there was anything she could do to increase Haley's resistance to bugs. "Wash your hands between handling kids," I suggested, the obvious advice, but Sondra assured me she was already doing that. Then I told her that glyconutrients have been shown to be helpful in improving immune function, and perhaps they could help Haley. On my advice, Sondra added a quarter-teaspoon (500 milligrams) once daily of a glyconutrient powder that contained arabinogalactans and aloe extracts to Haley's milk. (See the resources chapter for more information.) I told Sondra to double the dose should Haley start coming down with a cold. In the next six months, Haley had only one mild case of the sniffles.

*Suggested Use:* For adults: 1,000 milligrams in divided doses; double the dose if a cold is coming on. Before giving glyconutrients to your children, always consult your doctor. Infants and toddlers under two should be administered glyconutrients only under a doctor's supervision. Aloe and arabinogalactans mixture: 500 milligrams, once a day for children two to twelve; double the dose if a cold is coming on.

# Influenza

### POLYSACCHARIDE K

Flu vaccines promote specific immunity to particular strains of the influenza virus. Every year the flu virus alters genetically. That means your resistance last year will probably not protect you from this year's strain of the virus. Occasionally, scientists miscalculate which flu will prevail and produce the wrong vaccine. Because the flu makes millions of people sick every year—and kills many thousands—in worldwide epidemics, continued research on whether glyconutrients improve the resistance of human beings to the disease is important.

In one study, when scientists infected healthy mice with the influenza virus, the animals experienced an expected viral increase in their lungs. After a week, the level of virus began to decline. But in a subsequent experiment, before the scientists administered the flu virus, they gave the mice cyclophosphamide, a cancer drug that destroys rapidly dividing cells. On the upside, cyclophosphamide kills many kinds of cancer, but on the downside, those rapidly dividing cells include normal cells, like the hair on your head, and many immune cells as well, making those receiving it more susceptible to infection. Not surprisingly, the researchers found that in the second experiment, the cancer drug caused the level of flu virus to increase faster in the mice and stay higher for a longer time. But when researchers gave flu-infected mice the glyconutrient polysaccharide K followed by cyclophosphamide, the animals' ability to fight off the flu was restored.[4] These findings support an earlier study, again done on mice, in which glyconutrients also protected the animals against the flu.[5] Evidence from animal population studies also suggests that glyconutrients increase the effectiveness of certain flu vaccines.[6] That improved response might translate someday into more effective vaccinations and fewer required doses.

*Suggested Use:* Until human trials are conducted, we won't know if polysaccharide K fights the flu in humans, but the glyconutrient has been shown to boost immunity generally. To improve your overall immunity, you can try 1 to 6 grams of polysaccharide K daily, in divided doses. Start out slowly with a gram a day, divided into a dose in the morning and evening. In rare instances, polysaccharide K can cause darkening of the fingernails, a benign side effect. Other glyconutrients, including acemannan and yeast beta-glucans, may be useful in increasing resistance to the flu virus. Use 1 gram acemannan a day in divided doses and up to 100 milligrams beta-glucan once a day.

## Venereal Warts

### LENTINAN

Condyloma, better known as venereal warts, is a sexually transmitted viral disease. Sometimes the disease manifests as beady-looking growths, which appear in the external genital areas and around the anus and can enlarge to the size of a bunch of grapes in susceptible individuals; at other times, lesions appear on the cervix and are not visible externally. If the mother has an active infection, the infant can be infected as it travels through the birth canal. The virus also increases the risk of cervical cancer and is common in AIDS patients. While venereal warts can be burned off with chemicals or an ultracold probe (cryotherapy), the preferred method is laser therapy. Still, warts tend to recur again and again because those with the disorder suffer diminished cellular immunity.

Lentinan, a glyconutrient derived from the shiitake mushroom, enhances cellular immunity in condyloma patients. In a small 1999 study of thirty-six male and female patients, Chinese dermatologists demonstrated that treating individuals with lentinan orally, 12.5 milligrams twice a day, for six weeks before and two weeks after laser therapy decreased condyloma recurrence, as compared with controls, who received only laser treatment. Within ten weeks after treatment, two of the nineteen lentinan patients (10.5 percent) experienced a recurrence, versus eight of the seventeen controls (47 percent).[7] In addition, blood work showed that, unlike the control patients, the lentinan patients registered an increase in production of both helper T cells, critical in launching an effective immune response, and a protein called interleukin-2, which stimulates the production of additional helper T cells.

*Suggested Use:* If you have condyloma, see your doctor. For maintenance after laser or chemical therapy or cryotherapy, try 12.5 milligrams twice daily for a month, then taper off to 12.5 milligrams once a day. Injectable and intravenous lentinan are usually more effective than oral lentinan. Intravenous lentinan is available by prescription only and must be administered by a health-care professional. Serious side effects have occurred with intravenous lentinan, including fever, chills, back and leg pain, elevated liver enzymes, and anaphylaxis—a serious and potentially fatal allergic reaction. Doses are calculated according to the patient's weight and health status. (See the resources chapter for more information.)

## Herpes Viruses

### HERPES I AND II

Most of the glyconutrient research in herpes revolves around herpes I, or oral herpes; herpes II, or genital herpes; and cytomegalovirus, which does not usually cause significant disease in healthy adults and older children but can wreak havoc on the immunocompromised, especially those with AIDS, as well as the developing fetus.

About two-thirds of Americans are carriers of herpes I, which causes fever blisters in some people when they develop a cold or are stressed or run down. Of those infected, about half experience recurrences after the initial infection. Herpes II causes blisters on the genitals and can lead to cervical cancer. Oral and genital herpes infect by attaching to specific glycoproteins on the skin or mucous membranes of the mouth or genitals.[8] T cells and natural killer cells tend to keep recurrent herpes infections in check, but stress and illness decrease cellular immunity, resulting in the likelihood of more frequent and more severe episodes.

Very frequent outbreaks of any herpes virus suggest that something may be seriously wrong with the immune system.

## HERPES II: A PATIENT'S SUCCESS

Greg is a forty-year-old architect who's had genital herpes for twenty years. Until three years ago he suffered outbreaks of blisters on his penis about four times a year, with the eruption lasting about two weeks. The painful outbreaks usually started with an itching sensation that progressed to one or more blisters and then an open sore that took a week to heal. Unusual stress at work or at home usually preceded the outbreak. Prescription medicines, including the oral antiviral acyclovir and topical creams, often shortened the duration of the episode if started early enough. Greg also noticed that every time he ate lots of cashew nuts, the itching would resume. Arginine, an amino acid plentiful in nuts, has been implicated in herpes outbreaks.

In 1997, Greg began to take glyconutrients, including 3 grams of cordyceps daily as well as 1 gram of aloe and arabinogalactans daily, to improve his general health. (See the resources chapter for more information.) In the years since, he's had only one mild herpes outbreak. Occasionally he experiences mild genital itching, which resolves if he doubles his glyconutrient dose for a day or so.

*Suggested Use:* Until human studies are conducted, we won't know for sure if glyconutrients can help prevent herpes outbreaks. But to improve overall immune functioning, consider adding glyconutrients to your diet. Aloe and arabinogalactans: 500 milligrams to 1 gram a day, in divided doses. Cordyceps extracts or Cs-4: 3 to 6 grams daily. Do not add cordyceps extracts if you take blood thinners or have a bleeding disorder unless you are under a doctor's care, and the doctor has authorized you to take them.

In vitro studies have been done on herpes and glyconutrients, and the results look promising. Researchers reported suppression of herpes I—not due to the glyconutrients' killing of the virus but through the ability of the glyconutrients to stifle the virus's capacity to infect.[9] Similar results were reported by other scientists.[10] In a recent study, polysaccharide extracts from the reishi mushroom inhibited both herpes I and II in the test tube.[11] Combining the reishi polysaccharides with interferon worked synergistically to hamper both herpes I and II.

*Suggested Use:* It's too early to know if reishi extracts inhibit herpes viruses. But supplementing with reishi extracts may strengthen your immune system: 3 to 6 grams daily, in divided doses. Do not add reishi extracts if you take blood thinners or have a bleeding disorder unless you are under a doctor's care, and the doctor has authorized you to take them.

### CYTOMEGALOVIRUS

Cytomegalovirus has serious consequences for embryos and newborns, including major birth defects, miscarriages, mental retardation, small head size, low birth weight, and hepatitis. If animal studies are any indication, glyconutrients may someday help safeguard against this virus. Polysaccharide K, derived from the mushroom *Coriolus versicolor,* protects mice (for whom cytomegalovirus is deadly) from contracting the virus by increasing natural killer cell activity.[12] Nonetheless, pregnant women should *not* take polysaccharide K.

In time, as we get to understand more about them, dietary glyconutrients may become usable for pregnant women to support proper development of the fetus and provide some measure of protection from viruses and other harmful agents. For now, though, pregnant and nursing women should attempt to get the nutrients they need through a healthy diet.

*Suggested Use:* People with advanced HIV disease often develop cytomegalovirus infections. While scientists don't know if polysaccharide K will inhibit the infection in these patients, supplementing with polysaccharide K may confer improvement in immune status. Ask your doctor if you can try 3 to 6 grams daily, in divided doses. But start out slowly at 1 gram, and build gradually. For more on HIV, see chapter 12.

Your greatest defense for dealing with the thousands of viruses against which there are no cures or vaccines is to keep your inborn immune system defenses in good standing. Glyconutrients in your diet or as supplements may offer protection against viruses by boosting and optimizing the intelligence of your immune system.

## Chapter 6

# Treating Bacterial, Fungal, and Parasitic Infections

*Glyconutrients guard against chronic, recurrent ear infections in children and stave off infections from E. coli, yeast, and parasites.*

**A**t three weeks of age Colin was the youngest patient I had ever diagnosed with a bacterial ear infection. That was back in 1996. Over the next two years, he continued to come down with middle-ear infections, called otitis media, with alarming frequency. He received about twelve courses of antibiotics for infections in his first two years. On average, he developed an infection every couple of months. Placing tubes in his ears to allow the fluid to drain and removing his tonsils and adenoids didn't help. His mother, a social worker with a hectic work schedule, was at her wit's end. In 1998, when Colin was two years old, I started him on a mixture of aloe extracts and arabinogalactans (gum sugars found in plants), 500 milligrams daily, in two divided doses. Within three weeks, he was free of ear infections—and has remained so.

Since treating Colin, I've tried glyconutrient supplementation on four other children plagued with frequent ear infections, each of whom had each been taking six to ten courses of antibiotics a year. The results have been promising. Two children have remained symptom-free. One child did not come back for follow-up, and the fourth has had one ear infection in four months.

While a few case reports are not proof of anything, it would be just as foolish to discount them. After all, ear infections in children are a huge problem. The 30 million physician visits per year for ear infections cost some $4 billion annually to treat in the United States alone. Factoring in the costs in lost work time and family distress, that figure could easily be doubled. In addition, glyconutrients do not interfere with the effectiveness of antibiotics—unless the directions require that you take the antibiotics on an empty stomach—because unlike antibiotics, glyconutrients do not kill bacteria. Instead, glyconutrients empower the immune system to do its own killing.

## Mucosal Oligosaccharides: The First Line of Defense

Saccharides may have worked for Colin by preventing the bacteria responsible for his ear infections from securing a foothold. By binding to lectins—proteins on the walls of bacteria—protective saccharides called oligosaccharides prevent bacteria from attaching to the cells in the body. If the bacteria can't attach, they can't make you sick. Oligosaccharides (containing three to six monosaccharides) are found, among other places, in mucus, saliva, tears, urine, stomach acid, and sweat. Like an armed guard at a gate, oligosaccharides block the invasion of various germs, which may be coughed up in mucus or flushed away in the urine. Denied entry, the bugs are rendered noninfectious.

Scientific and anecdotal evidence suggest that supplementing your diet with glyconutrients improves immunity, enabling the body to respond more quickly and more specifically to eliminate pathogens that do gain entry. Deficiencies in essential saccharides may cause your cells to produce abnormal glycoproteins, making infections more likely.

In 1996, in the medical journal *Lancet*, researchers Zopf and Roth reported that in animal studies oligosaccharides have been effective against several bacteria, including *E. coli*, *Bordetella pertussis* (the pathogen responsible for whooping cough), *Streptococcus pneumoniae* (a strep bug that causes pneumonia), and *Helicobacter pylori* (the causative agent for some peptic ulcers).[1] Interestingly, in the age of antibiotic-resistant bugs, oligosaccharides hold particular promise because they are unlikely to cause resistance: unlike antibiotics, they don't kill bacteria directly.

Some people have more abundant, more diverse, and more protective oligosaccharides in their mucus than others. As explained by biophysicists at the Weizmann Institute of Science in Rehovot, Israel, adhesion of bacteria and the effects that result vary not only from species to species but among animals of the same species.[2] Certainly genetics and perhaps diet account for the differences within the same species.

In addition, certain bacteria fancy certain sites: *E. coli*, for instance, take to the bladder and kidneys but aren't keen on the upper respiratory tract, whereas strep has a penchant for the upper respiratory tract but not much proclivity for the bladder.[3] Wherever the bacteria colonize, glyconutrient supplements provide the raw materials necessary for creating a first-class defense system of saccharides and oligosaccharides, bolstering the body's defense.

*Suggested Use:* Your doctor should approve any glyconutrients for children. Glyconutrients should not be given to any children under age two unless under a doctor's supervision. For children ages two to twelve years, the suggested dose for your doctor to approve is 500 milligrams of aloe and arabinogalactans, in two divided doses with water a half-hour before meals. In general, children two and older should take *half* the manufacturer's *lowest recommended dose* for adults. For more information, see chapter 3.

# Other Bacterial Infections

### E. COLI

The bacterium *Escherichia coli* has garnered a lot of press from its contamination of hamburger and water, which led to several deaths in the United States a couple of years ago. A normal inhabitant of the large intestine, *E. coli* instigates trouble if it ventures outside, causing urinary tract infections, kidney disease, and even death. Toxins produced by certain strains of *E. coli* can damage platelets and red blood cells, causing them to clump together, producing in rare cases a potentially fatal disease called hemolytic-uremic syndrome. This syndrome can instigate damage to multiple organs and kidney failure.

Israeli researchers performed an experiment on mice in which bladder infections were induced with *E. coli*.[4] When particular combinations of mannose saccharides were injected along with the *E. coli*, the scientists found that the sugars' presence reduced bacterial growth and infectivity. Also encouraging is that in vitro studies indicate that the same protection holds true for human cells.[5] Perhaps one day doctors will prescribe glyconutrients prophylactically to individuals who suffer from frequent urinary tract infections.

*Suggested Use:* If you have symptoms of a bladder infection, see your doctor immediately, as you will need antibiotics. Left untreated, bladder infections can spread to the kidneys and cause permanent damage. Until human studies are done, we won't know if mannose and other saccharides inhibit urinary tract infections in people. If you suffer from frequent bladder infections, you may want to boost your immunity with powdered aloe extracts, which are rich in mannose: 250 milligrams one to three times daily.

### MENINGITIS

*Neisseria meningitidis* is a highly aggressive bacterium that can cause a rapidly fatal form of meningitis. Occasionally, schools in the United States close because a student becomes ill with this highly contagious infection, which thrives in crowded settings like schools and military barracks. As with other communicable diseases, why some people exposed contract meningitis and others don't is still a mystery. However, British scientists have found that individuals who come down with *Neisseria* infections are up to six and a half times more likely to have inherited from both parents a genetic variant of a mannose-binding lectin that makes them more susceptible to infection.[6]

It's not known at this time if supplementing with mannose polysaccharides will help guard against meningitis. If you have been exposed to meningitis, see your doctor *immediately* for treatment and prophylactic antibiotics. Do *not* take glyconutrients to treat meningitis.

## Fungal Infections

Animal studies indicate that glyconutrients are protective against yeast infections in immunosuppressed mice. In these mice, the glyconutrient polysaccharide K, for instance, heightens the immune response against the yeast and prolongs their lives.[7] Furthermore, researchers have found that acemannan, an aloe polysaccharide, prevented the infectious yeast from adhering to the gastrointestinal tract in mice inoculated with the yeast. The investigators postulated that acemannan may bind to the mucous membranes in the intestinal tract, blocking the yeast's attachment.[8]

In 1997, researchers tested the activity of macrophages incubated in the glyconutrient acemannan against yeast and compared the results with macrophages not exposed to the aloe extract.[9] Macrophages exposed to acemannan for ten minutes resulted in more than a third of the yeast organisms being killed, as compared with 0 to 5 percent in the controls. When the macrophages were incubated for sixty minutes, the results were even more impressive: some 98 percent of the yeast organisms were killed by the glyconutrient-treated macrophages, as compared with, again, only 0 to 5 percent in controls.

## FUNGAL INFECTIONS: A PATIENT'S SUCCESS

Deborah is a thirty-two-year-old physician who's suffered from re-current vaginal yeast infections for five years. *Candida albicans,* the organism that causes yeast infections in human beings, is a normal inhabitant of the large intestine, where the fungus is kept in check by our immune systems and the healthful bacteria of the gut. When an imbalance occurs in our immune systems, yeast may overgrow in the gut, throat, vagina, or skin. Occasional yeast infections are rarely a cause for concern. Some otherwise healthy women are prone to vaginal yeast infections, and some babies develop diaper rash on their bottoms or thrush in their throats. Most yeast infections can be relatively minor and easily treated, but in people with weakened immune systems—very premature babies and bone-marrow transplant recipients, for instance—yeast infections can be life threatening. Individuals with AIDS, cancer, diabetes, chronic fatigue syndrome, and Gulf War syndrome and those taking steroids are similarly prone to yeast infections.

Deborah told me she didn't have any predisposing conditions to explain her frequent yeast infections, and her general health was good. She noted, however, that her occasional use of antibi-otics for bladder infections invariably brought on a yeast infection. (Antibiotics kill off healthful bacteria that keep yeast in check.) In the past, she usually had treated her yeast infec-tions with yeast-killing vaginal creams, including Mycostatin and Monistat, and the infections resolved—only to recur.

Deborah heard about my interest in glyconutrients and their effects on immunity, so she sought my advice. I suggested a mix-ture of aloe extracts and arabinogalactans, 1,000 milligrams a day, in divided doses, and they worked better than she had hoped: She has been free of yeast infections for ten months (see the resources section for more information).

*Suggested Use:* If you are experiencing recurrent yeast in-fections, it is prudent to get a medical work-up to rule out an underlying condition that may be responsible. Once serious illness has been excluded, consult with your doctor about supplementing with glyconutrients. From animal and test-tube studies, we know that aloe is effective in killing yeast. But until human studies are done, we won't know if this regimen will work for everyone. Taking aloe and arabinogalactans, however, is a good way to boost immunity, at 500 milligrams once or twice a day.

## Parasitic Infections

In a study on mice at Israel's Weizmann Institute of Science, scientists found that polysaccharides obtained from beta-glucans suppressed the progression of a parasitic infection from *Leishmania*, a protozoa transmitted to animals and humans by sand flies, which results in fevers, liver and spleen enlargement, ulcerative skin conditions, and wasting.[10] Without treatment, death occurs within two years in most symptomatic individuals. Variants of the disease occur in India, China, Africa, southern Russia, and South and Central America.

Arabinogalactans are effective against *Leishmania* as well. In 1989, German researchers found that arabinogalactans from the popular herb *Echinacea* increase the release of parasite-killing free radicals within macrophages, resulting in enhanced killing of the parasite.[11] In vitro studies suggest that maitake mushrooms may be valuable in fighting the parasite that causes malaria.[12]

Another parasitic infection called toxocarosis, caused by the parasite *Toxocara*, is commonly found in dogs, cats, wolves, and foxes and can be spread to humans. The parasite migrates throughout the body, particularly affecting the lungs, eyes, heart, liver, and spleen. In an animal study, researchers induced a serious infection in mice, but polysaccharide beta-glucans given to the mice resulted in a significant decrease in the parasite's ability to migrate in the host.[13]

*Suggested Use:* If you believe you may have a parasitic infection, see your doctor. Excellent medications exist to treat parasites, sometimes in only a few doses.

Should you be traveling to areas where the aforementioned parasites are endemic, taking mushroom or yeast beta-glucans, or rice, oat, or barley brans, which also contain beta-glucans, is a good idea to improve your overall health. For rice, oat, or barley brans, read labels carefully. To enhance flavor, some manufacturers add sweetener, which diabetics and those watching their weight should avoid. Follow the manufacturer's suggestions or your doctor's advice. For reasons that aren't currently understood, *Echinacea* loses its efficacy with prolonged use. Take the manufacturer's recommended dose. As an immune booster, *Echinacea* works well in cycles of two weeks on and two weeks off.

To enhance immunity, you can also try mushroom extracts from cordyceps, shiitake, or reishi: 1 to 3 grams a day, in divided doses. Do not add cordyceps or reishi extracts if you take a blood-thinner or have a bleeding disorder unless you are under a doctor's care, and the doctor has authorized you to take them.

## Chapter 7

# Alleviating Allergies, Asthma, and Other Pulmonary Diseases

---

*What is different about the way nonallergic people harmlessly handle substances that cause problems in allergic people and asthmatics? Saccharides may be key.*

I once asked an asthma researcher why it is that most of us never wheeze or suffer other symptoms that asthmatics do, although we all breathe the same air, eat more or less the same kinds of foods, and are exposed to similar stressors. He was stumped. He couldn't give me an answer because it wasn't the kind of question that he'd normally ask. His job was to evaluate drugs that suppress asthma symptoms and improve the patient's quality of life. Like most scientists, he was focused on what makes us sick and how to manage the illness, not how to keep us well or get us well. His job is a prime example of establishment, or allopathic, Western medicine, which I also call "rescue medicine."

The medical establishment for too long has overlooked why people are well. What is different in the way asthmatics and nonasthmatics handle the same pollen or perfume? Why are these agents harmless to some and disease-inducing in others?

It's important for our lungs to live amicably with sundry environmental antigens because chronic inflammation interferes with the effectiveness of breathing, the most elemental act of living. Many scientists believe that certain factors in the mucus in nonallergic individuals help protect them from developing full-blown immunological reactions to pedestrian nuisances. To understand abnormality, however, we first have to examine "normality."

Well-functioning saccharides are part of the answer to normality. We know that protective saccharides in the mucus and breast milk block bacteria, viruses, and parasites from landing, rendering these pathogens powerless to infect. You could think of them as the fighter planes of your immune system, taking out the enemy before they've had a chance to settle in and cause damage.[1] There is evidence that saccharides prevent allergens from securing a foothold as well.

In controlled studies, saccharides have been shown to be efficacious against allergies and asthma, as well as pneumonia, tuberculosis, and bronchitis. This is good news because asthma causes two to three thousand deaths per year in the United States, and the incidence is increasing. According to the Asthma and Allergy Foundation of America, of the 17 million Americans who suffer from asthma, 5.5 million are kids under eighteen: that's more than double from 1980. An estimated 60 million Americans suffer from allergies, which constitute the sixth leading cause of chronic disease in the United States. Dust mites, cockroaches, mold, pollen, animal dander, car emissions, and cigarette smoke are big offenders. Diseased lungs react differently to the offending antigen than healthy lungs do, generating free radicals that exacerbate lung inflammation.

## Allergies

The key to understanding allergy, including asthma, is immunoglobulin E (IgE), one of a class of five major antibodies; IgG, IgA, IgM, and IgD are the other four. Normally, the lungs, skin, and mucous membranes launch an attack with IgE against infestations—insects, worms, chiggers, and flukes—but not against viruses and bacterial infections. While IgE, along with the other four antibodies in this class, is a glycoprotein, it behaves differently from the other four: the other antibodies are free-floating, but the codependent IgE attaches to what are called mast cells, which release histamine to subdue the offending pathogen. (The body is prepared to suffer some collateral damage to restrain parasites from infiltrating.) This is why we take *anti*histamines to counter the watery eyes, sneezing, and wheezing that histamines bring on.

But people with allergies are different from those without them. Allergic people produce IgE against such harmless items as house dust and cat dander. For some reason, while the rest of humanity produces IgG or IgM antibodies against these substances, allergic individuals generate more IgE. When the body unleashes big-gun immune-system weapons against pedestrian nuisances like pollen or peanut butter or the sting of a bee, the result can be the benign misery of a stuffed nose and watery eyes, or the life-threatening consequences of a severe asthma attack.

Before coming to America, I lived and practiced medicine in Cameroon, Africa, where the incidence of asthma and allergies is low. One of the theories advanced for this phenomenon is that the much higher infectious disease load in that country propels people's immune system in a nonallergic direction. Indeed, many scientists now believe that the decline in infectious diseases in industrialized countries has altered the way in which the immune system reacts. For instance, a 1997 Japanese study suggests that a higher incidence of tuberculosis correlates with reduced allergy occurrence.[2] Here in the United States we've become too clean and healthy for our own good—and the result is an overreaction to harmless substances. The question is, what can be done about it?

Avoidance is one solution. If crabmeat makes you break out in hives, by all means steer clear of it. If cat dander causes you to sneeze and your eyes to itch, avoid cats. Reducing exposure makes practical sense, and it works. But sometimes limiting exposure is difficult or impossible, particularly if pollens, grasses, and molds trigger your asthma or allergies. What helps are antihistamines, steroids, and a fairly new class of drugs that inhibits potent mediators of inflammation called leukotrienes, though the effects of all three are temporary. Allergy shots are another approach: the allergic person is injected with a very dilute mixture of the substance that provokes the allergic response—the purpose of which is to enable greater tolerance to the allergen or to instruct the immune system to make non-IgE antibodies.

Glyconutrients also help. There is substantial evidence that some glyconutrients can reduce the amount of IgE in the blood, thereby diminishing symptoms caused by IgE overproduction. In Cameroon, we ate a polysaccharide called chitin (pronounced KI·tin) virtually every day. Composed of the essential sugar N-acetylglucosamine, it's present in mushrooms and in the shells of crustaceans, including shrimp, krill, and crabs. One excellent source of chitin is *njanga*, a species of tiny shrimp caught off the coast of Africa; they're so small they're not worth shelling. Instead, they're smoke-dried to crisp perfection over blazing mangrove wood, and then—shells and all—crushed into powder and used as a condiment in many savory dishes.

In a controlled study in 2000, researchers found that when mice with induced ragweed allergy received finely ground chitin for three days before and three days after being injected with ragweed pollen, they experienced significantly lower levels of allergy-mediating IgE, as well as higher IgG levels and significantly fewer eosinophils (white blood cells produced in the allergic response) in their lungs, compared with allergic controls, who received a placebo.[3]

Other glyconutrients also help fight the overproduction of histamine. Researchers have reported that extracts of the reishi mushroom reduce the release of histamine in animals.[4] And ling zhi-8, one of reishi's glycoprotein extracts, has been shown to prevent fatal allergic reactions in animals.[5] Several other reishi mushroom compounds—including oleic acid (an unsaturated fatty acid) and ganoderic acids (similar in composition to steroids)—while not saccharides, also inhibit histamine release in rats.[6, 7]

*Suggested Use:* Glyconutrients should *never* be used as a treatment *during* an allergic or asthmatic episode; they're for preventive care only. They are also not a substitute for established preventive or maintenance care of asthma.

Pure chitin is available only to commercial vendors, but you can make your own. (See the resources chapter for two of my favorite chitin recipes.) Chitosan is chitin modified by acid and alkali. Unlike chitin, chitosan can bind fat and is used for weight loss (see chapter 13). Follow directions on the manufacturer's label (see the resources chapter for sources). Caution: If you are allergic to shellfish, do *not* try chitin or chitosan, as both are made from shellfish.

Because the reishi extract studies on histamine release have been conducted only on animals, we don't know if the effects apply to humans, but supplementing with reishi extracts may improve your overall health. Follow your doctor's recommendations and the instructions on the manufacturer's label. Do not take reishi extracts if you take a blood thinner or have a bleeding disorder unless under a doctor's care.

## Asthma, Bronchitis, and Chronic Obstructive Pulmonary Disease (COPD)

Chronic asthma causes lung swelling and thick secretions within the asthmatic lung—and as a result, the lungs take in less oxygen. Asthma can lead to permanent lung damage and chronic obstructive pulmonary disease (COPD). Breathing becomes chronically labored and shallow, particularly on exertion. Patients often use bronchodilators to open up their airways and anti-inflammatories to reduce inflammation. In severe cases, patients are put on oxygen.

Scientists in a two-part comprehensive overview of cordyceps and its extract Cs-4 presented several compelling human studies on the effects of the glyconutrients on diseases of the lungs, including asthma. Among them is a 1995 Chinese trial in which thirty-five elderly COPD patients took three grams of the cordyceps extract Cs-4 for three weeks.[8] Participants reported improvements in appetite, vitality, and pulmonary symptoms and decreases in cough, wheezing, and phlegm. The researchers also noted a rise in the antioxidant superoxide dismutase (SOD) in the patients. SOD fights the free radicals that are part of a vicious cycle in which the inflammation in asthmatic lungs causes the body to produce more free radicals, which in turn stokes the inflammation already present.[9] In another controlled Chinese study, researchers found that 83 percent of patients with respiratory diseases who received Cs-4 treatment for one month responded, compared with 40 percent of the controls.[10] The Cs-4 patients reported that they felt stronger physically. In fact, by the end of the study some were able to jog a tenth of a mile.

In animal studies, glyconutrients have been shown to mitigate coughs and serve as an expectorant, increasing secretions and allowing mucus to be coughed up from the lungs more easily. A Chinese study concluded that mice given Cs-4 along with cough-inducing ammonia coughed two-thirds less frequently than the controls.[11] And, in an experiment on guinea pigs, Cs-4 relaxed tracheal muscles to prevent the spasms caused by histamine.[12] Scientists in 1986 reported that in albino rats with induced bronchitis, daily injections of reishi extracts not only reduced coughing and increased expectoration but also induced regeneration of the cells of the bronchial epithelium, which covers the surface of the bronchial tubes.[13]

Aloe extracts have also been shown to be effective. In a small study of thirty-three adult asthmatics, aloe increased the ability of white blood cells to engulf foreign bodies.[14] However, for patients concomitantly administered steroids, the aloe was not helpful. *Patients with asthma or other pulmonary illnesses should never discontinue steroids without conferring with their physician.*

Glyconutrients can also induce cellular healing in pulmonary diseases. Reishi mushrooms are effective in treating chronic bronchitis, particularly in older adults. In one study of more than 2,000 patients, Chinese researchers found that reishi extracts brought significant improvement in 60 to 90 percent of the participants.[15]

*Suggested Use:* Glyconutrients should *never* be used as a treatment during an allergic or asthmatic episode; they're for preventive care only, as an adjunct to standard therapy and to be taken only with your doctor's knowledge and approval. Discuss with your doctor taking cordyceps extract or Cs-4: 3 to 6 grams daily, in divided doses, as a supplement to your regular medication.

Alternative supplements include powdered, stabilized aloe extracts, 250 milligrams two to three times a day; and reishi extracts, 3 to 6 grams daily, in divided doses. Do not take cordyceps or reishi extracts if you take a blood thinner or have a bleeding disorder unless under a doctor's care.

If you combine two glyconutrients, cut the dose for each by half; if you combine three, cut the dose for each by two-thirds, and so on. Start with one glyconutrient at a time, and build slowly. Saccharides help prevent allergens from securing a foothold in the body, heading off allergic and asthmatic reactions. Glyconutrients also reduce the amount of IgE in the blood, thereby easing allergic symptoms caused by IgE overproduction and reducing the inflammation characteristic of the asthmatic lung. Glyconutrients fight free radicals by generating antioxidants. Finally, some studies indicate that glyconutrients mitigate coughs and serve as an expectorant, increasing secretions that more easily allow the lungs to expel mucus.

## OTHER RESPIRATORY DISEASES: A PATIENT'S SUCCESS

Fifty-one-year-old Victoria owns a chain of clothing stores and tools around her neighborhood in a silver Hummer. If you saw this vital, physically active woman today, you'd have difficulty believing what she went through a few years ago.

In early 1997, Victoria came down with what she thought was the flu. She got better but developed a persistent dry cough and shortness of breath. She was put on oxygen. Surgeons biopsied Victoria's lung in November of 1997, and pathologists made the diagnosis: bronchiolitis obliterans with organizing pneumonia—BOOP, for short, as it is known, even by doctors. BOOP is not the sort of condition diagnosed at a walk-in visit to a physician's office. The disorder hits men and women equally in their forties and fifties and shares features both of viral pneumonia and of autoimmune disease. It's idiopathic, which means no one knows what causes it. It has nothing to do with smoking. What happens is that scar and inflamed tissue form in the bronchial tubes, so that over time they become heavy and stiff, making breathing labored and difficult. Doctors prescribed a steroid called prednisone—a medicine that results in recovery in two-thirds of those treated. After six months of treatment Victoria's condition stabilized, but she continued to need oxygen.

In the fall of 1999, Victoria experienced pain and trouble breathing and was rushed to the hospital, where she was placed in intensive care. Doctors performed a tracheostomy (surgery to make an opening in the windpipe), and Victoria was started on a ventilator. Her condition continued to deteriorate; she developed a fever and a life-threatening bacterial blood infection called sepsis. Antibiotics eradicated the blood infection, and Victoria's holistic physician started her on powdered aloe extracts (250 milligrams three times daily) and arabinogalactans (2 grams daily, in divided doses; see the resources section). Within six weeks Victoria was breathing on her own.

By twelve weeks Victoria started rehabilitation. Four weeks later she was discharged. Today she's off oxygen entirely and her lungs function normally. She still suffers residual nerve pain from the illness, but she is well otherwise. She continues to take glyconutrients daily.

*Suggested Use for Boosting Immunity:* Supplementing with Victoria's regimen of aloe extracts and arabinogalactans daily may prove helpful for overall immunity. Stabilized, powdered aloe extracts, 250 milligrams, two to three times daily, and arabinogalactans, 1 to 3 grams daily, in divided doses.

## Chapter 8

# Healing Skin Disorders, Burns, and Wounds

*Treating psoriasis, pemphigoid, seborrheic dermatitis, poison ivy, burns, and wounds with glyconutrients.*

Skin diseases vary from the short-lived and benign to the chronic and life-threatening. But whatever the prognosis, skin disorders can diminish self-esteem, sometimes wounding the soul more than the skin. In his 1989 autobiography, *Self-Consciousness: Memoirs,* novelist John Updike, who suffers from psoriasis, confided that he became a writer primarily so that he could avoid facing people every day. "Because of my skin," he explains, "I counted myself out of any of those jobs—salesman, teacher, financier, movie star—that demand being presentable. What did that leave? Becoming a craftsman of some sort, closeted and unseen—perhaps a cartoonist or a writer, a worker in ink who can hide himself and send out a surrogate presence, a signature that multiplies even while it conceals."[1]

Nevertheless, for Updike the illness remained torturous, a source of unremitting rumination: "Psoriasis keeps you thinking. Strategies of concealment ramify, and self-examination is endless. You are forced to the mirror again and again; psoriasis compels narcissism, if we can suppose a Narcissus who did not like what he saw. In certain lights, your face looks passable; in slightly different other lights, not. . . . I cannot pass a reflecting surface on the street without glancing in, in hopes that I have somehow changed."[2]

## Psoriasis

Many researchers believe psoriasis is an autoimmune disease, in which the immune system turns on itself, attacking its own cells, which it's supposed to protect. Psoriasis is associated with arthritis and does respond to immunosuppressive drugs. In people who have the disease, which tends to be inherited and affects about 2 percent of the population, the immune system's T cells in the skin malfunction, and the result is inflammation and excessive reproduction of skin cells. The condition can be limited to a few patches or can cover the entire body.

### ALOE VERA

*Aloe vera* gel has been used for centuries to treat inflammatory skin conditions. Rich in saccharides, the glyconutrient is effective in treating psoriasis. Mannose polysaccharides are responsible for the healing properites of aloe. *Aloe vera* gel must be used shortly after the leaf is harvested, or stabilized by a freeze-drying process. Buyers beware: If the aloe product is not stabilized, don't buy it. *Unstabilized* aloe gel has been exposed to air for several hours and has become degraded, losing its healing properties. Not only does unstabilized gel not work, it has been found to *hinder* healing.[3, 4]

Researchers at Malmo University Hospital in Sweden tested a topical *Aloe vera* cream versus a placebo cream in a double-blind study of 60 patients ages eighteen to fifty with chronic psoriasis. Patients were examined weekly for sixteen weeks, followed by a year of monthly follow-ups. No adverse symptoms were reported in either group, and no one dropped out of the study. By the end of the trial, the *Aloe vera* cream resulted in a remission in 83 percent of patients, versus the placebo remission rate of only 6.6 percent.[5]

*Suggested Use:* When applying *Aloe vera* for the first time, dab on a little in an inconspicuous spot on your leg or arm and wait twenty-four hours to see if you develop an allergic reaction. Should skin become red and itchy or should you develop hives, discontinue use. If you find you are not allergic, apply stabilized topical *Aloe vera* gel several times to the affected area, keeping the skin moist.

If the affected area is extensive, take 250 milligrams of *Aloe vera* stabilized powder two to four times a day with a glass of water a half-hour before meals. The oral form will take longer to work (from a week to a few months), but results over the long term may be better.

## PEMPHIGOID: A PATIENT'S SUCCESS

Sherry is a fifty-year-old woman with a history of diabetes and hypothyroidism. In the winter of 1997 she developed several blisters on her scalp that turned into sores and then coalesced to form a large, painful wound four inches wide and eight inches long. A dermatologist diagnosed pemphigoid, an autoimmune skin disease that results in painful blisters and ulcers that heal slowly—or not at all. The mainstay treatment is steroids; antibiotics and chemotherapy agents like cyclophosphamide are also used. Sherry's doctor prescribed steroids and cyclosphosphamide. Occasionally the lesions got infected, and then she'd add antibiotics to the mix. For the next year and a half she continued with this debilitating treatment protocol.

In June 1998, in an attempt to improve her overall health, Sherry added glyconutrients to her regimen. She took 250 milligrams of stabilized aloe powder and 1.5 grams of arabinogalactans twice a day, before breakfast and dinner. (See the resources section for more information.) Sherry noted a slight improvement in her skin after four months—but a waxing and waning with autoimmune diseases is natural, so she wasn't convinced her small improvement had anything to do with saccharides. Then, suddenly, between the fourth and fifth months, the healing process accelerated like time-lapse photography, and the pemphigoid healed completely.

Interestingly, at the same time, Sherry's requirement for insulin reduced drastically from 150 units to 50 units a day, and her doctors also lowered her dose of thyroid medication. When I last spoke to Sherry, in January 2000, she had been weaned off insulin completely, managing her diabetes by diet alone. She also reported feeling more energetic. Her dermatologist, she said, was impressed by her improvement and encouraged her to "Keep doing what you're doing"—doctor-speak for: "I don't understand this alternative stuff, but it seems to be helping, so carry on with it."

Anecdotes like these are not proof that glyconutrients will cure pemphigoid—or even that they cured Sherry. Sometimes autoimmune diseases spontaneously disappear. But when we combine stories like Sherry's with the long history of saccharide use as well as with recent animal and human studies, they add up to compelling grounds to fund larger studies.

*Suggested Use:* No human or animal studies have been done on pemphigoid and glyconutrients. If standard medications aren't controlling the skin disorder, consider consulting your doctor about trying glyconutrients, including Sherry's regimen. Also consider adding glyconutrient-rich mushrooms to your diet, including maitake, shiitake, and oyster.

## Seborrheic Dermatitis

The inflammatory skin condition seborrheic dermatitis is thought to be caused by the body's overreaction to *Pityrosporum* yeasts and to products that break down oil.[6] Scaling, crusty yellow patches, redness, and itching on the scalp and face result. Aloe has proved to be an effective treatment. In a 1999 double-blind study, dermatologists treated forty-four seborrheic dermatitis patients with a topical *Aloe vera* emulsion.[7] After the trial, the doctors reported that 58 percent of the aloe patients improved, versus 15 percent of controls. Specifically, scaliness, itching, and the number of afflicted sites diminished. Redness, however, did not.

*Suggested Use:* For moderate or severe seborrheic dermatitis, see your doctor. For mild dermatitis, apply stabilized *Aloe vera* gel to the affected area several times a day, keeping the area moist. When applying *Aloe vera* for the first time, dab on a little in an inconspicuous spot on your leg or arm and wait twenty-four hours to see if you have an allergic reaction.

If skin becomes red and itchy or you develop hives, discontinue use. If itching and scaliness worsen, stop the aloe and consult your doctor. If the affected area is extensive, take 250 milligrams of stabilized *Aloe vera* powder two to four times a day with a glass of water a half-hour before meals. The oral form will take longer to work (from a week to a few months), but results over the long-term may be better.

## POISON IVY: A PATIENT'S SUCCESS

In July 1999, twelve-year-old Jonathan came to see me with his mother. This was the second time in two months that he had contracted poison ivy. Jonathan is an active kid, always getting into things, and the tiny red blisters on his arms and legs were cramping his style and making him miserable. I was wary of starting him on his second course of steroids, as previously he had needed them for ten days. Instead, I gave his mother an over-the-counter skin gel containing aloe polysaccharides and asked her to apply the emulsion several times a day, making sure that the skin remained coated with gel. In addition, I prescribed an antihistamine called Atarax, which causes drowsiness. But as anyone who's ever had a severe case of poison ivy can attest, antihistamines seldom provide significant relief from the incessant itch. A case in point was Jonathan: Although the antihistamine had helped him sleep during his last bout with poison ivy, it hadn't stopped him from scratching. He had better luck with the *Aloe vera*: twenty-four hours after it was applied, the itching was just about gone, and one week later when I saw him for follow-up, the lesions had healed.

*Suggested Use:* For moderate or severe poison ivy, see your doctor. For mild poison ivy, cleanse the affected area with warm water, pat dry, and apply stabilized *Aloe vera* gel several times a day, keeping the area moist. If itching and discomfort do not improve or they worsen, stop the aloe and consult your doctor.

When applying *Aloe vera* for the first time, it's a good idea to dab on a little in an inconspicuous spot on your leg or arm and wait twenty-four hours to see if you have an allergic reaction. If skin becomes red and itchy or you develop hives, discontinue use.

## Burn Healing

Healing begins with the very first response to a traumatic event as the clotting system and the immune system are mobilized. Once the acute crisis is under control, cells begin to migrate into the traumatized area to replace the damaged tissue; new blood vessels also begin to grow. If the injury has caused a skin defect, the body appears to know exactly where to lay down new skin.

Like any trauma to the skin, a burn is a forceful removal of tissue. The body faces the challenge of resisting or reversing infection and dehydration and then replacing the tissue. In humans, stabilized *Aloe vera* increased skin formation and decreased healing time in burn victims. In one study of twenty-seven patients with second-degree burns, those burns treated with topical *Aloe vera* healed in twelve days, versus eighteen days for control patients who received standard preparations.[8]

For a few days to weeks after laser resurfacing of the skin for wrinkles or acne, the skin may be pink or red, as if it's sustained a mild burn. In a controlled study at New York's St. Luke's Roosevelt Hospital at Columbia University, nineteen patients who had the procedure were randomly assigned to receive one of two skin dressings: a standard dressing used to reduce moisture loss, or a bovine cartilage ointment, rich in saccharides. Healing was

more rapid in the bovine cartilage group, with swelling and redness resolving more quickly.[9]

*Suggested Use for Burns:* For large or serious burns, see a physician immediately. For small, minor burns, immediately apply
cold water or ice for a few minutes, then lightly pat dry and apply
aloe gel several times a day, keeping the area moist. Break open a
leaf from an *Aloe vera* plant and use the inner clear gel to coat the
affected area, or use stabilized gel. Cover with gauze if you're going out; otherwise, leave the area uncovered.

*Suggested Use Following Laser Resurfacing:* Before applying aloe
or bovine cartilage ointment to your skin, consult your physician,
as allergic reactions may occur. When applying either for the first
time, dab on a little in an inconspicuous spot on your leg or arm
and wait twenty-four hours to see if you develop an allergic reaction. If skin becomes red and itchy or you develop hives, discontinue use.

### PREMATURE INFANT SKIN: A PATIENT'S SUCCESS

Premature babies born before thirty weeks of gestation tend to
have delicate, gelatinous, paper-thin skin that behaves as if it has
sustained a severe burn; it's like a leaky sieve, losing fluids and
breaking down easily. In April 1999, a baby named Henry was
born at twenty-five weeks at Our Lady of Lourdes Medical Center
in Camden, New Jersey, weighing just 1.4 pounds. Very premature
infants like Henry are usually hooked up to a ventilator and given
antibiotics and IV fluids. We coated Henry's skin with Aquaphor
lotion, to give some measure of protection from fluid loss. In addition, we covered his little bed with a layer of Saran Wrap to create a moist environment. Nevertheless, Henry, like many premies,
suffered skin problems in the form of abrasions and bruises. On
his second day of life he suffered breakdown of skin on his buttocks. The tissues appeared black and nonviable on a large segment of his buttocks on the third day. We cleaned the skin with
saline and applied antibiotic cream. Still, his skin continued to
break down. His condition was grave, but we were all rooting for
him and trying to find ways to help him.

On the fifth day, out of desperation and with the hospital's consent, I tried something new: a topical gel blend of aloe and arabinogalactans—the latter from the larch tree. (See resources chapter for more information.) The next day the baby's condition stabilized, and within forty-eight hours there was evidence of healing as the edges of the wound began to develop a healthy pink color. By the tenth day, the buttocks were pink and healthy, having healed completely and without scarring. Henry was weaned off the ventilator over the next couple of months and was discharged three months after he was born, ready at last to begin his life.

## Wound Healing

Whatever the species, wounds typically heal more slowly in older beings. This slowdown has been attributed to reduced immune functioning, lack of enough nutrients in the diet, and prolonged free-radical damage to the body's tissues. In diabetics, the body is unable to marshal the resources to form a decent scar and the wound remains open. Researchers have discovered that acemannan, the polysaccharide extracted from *Aloe vera*, accelerates wound healing in aged rats—so much so that the wounds of old, treated rats heal *faster* than those of young, untreated rats.[10]

*Aloe vera* hastens wound healing in animals whether given orally or used topically. In one study, investigators induced wounds near the vertebral column of mice.[11] Some of the mice then received *Aloe vera* in their drinking water for two months, while the controls received plain water. Another group of mice received topical aloe cream mixed with Eucerin hand cream, whereas the controls got only the Eucerin. After two months, the scientists recorded that the wounds in the mice given oral or topical aloe had become smaller and had healed better than the wounds of the controls. The investigators theorized that aloe increased oxygen and blood flow to injured areas by dilating capillaries, which could be particularly important in diabetes, where vascular circulation is impaired. Other studies suggest that aloe facilitates healing by jump-starting the immune response, activating the macrophages by boasting nitric oxide levels.[12]

When researchers in India conducted a wound study on rats treated with aloe, they found an increased turnover of collagen—the fibrous protein in skin and other connective tissue—at the site of the wound.[13] And in a comparative study on guinea pigs, *Aloe vera* gel extract was superior to the topical antimicrobial agent Silvadene as well as salicylic cream (an aspirin-like compound) or plain gauze dressing in treating burns. The wounds of the animals treated with aloe healed in an average of thirty days, whereas the average healing time for all the other guinea pigs was fifty days.[14] In addition, Silvadene and the stabilized aloe product decreased bacterial counts in the wounds equally.

Recent animal studies suggest that topical antibacterial salves and creams used on burns and wounds, while effective against microbes, are also toxic to cells that foster wound repair, and actually impede healing.[15] Aloe, however, has the ability both to decrease bacterial counts *and* facilitate wound repair. Evidence from animal studies indicates that aloe and other glyconutrients reduce postoperative infections and recovery time after surgery, as well as reduce the size of scars and improve their cosmetic appearance,[16] which may make glyconutrients particularly useful after plastic or reconstructive surgery.

Researchers at the Pennsylvania College of Podiatric Medicine and other institutions have shown that aloe is a potent anti-inflammatory as well.[17] Inflammation is one of the body's cruder responses to trauma and other kinds of damage. Although some inflammation is necessary for healing, it also leads to increased pain, swelling, and the shutting off of small blood vessels that bring nutrients and immune cells into the damaged site. Remarkably, glyconutrients simultaneously reduce inflammation while hastening healing. In addition, scientists have discovered that while steroids reduce the tensile strength of wounds in animals (tensile strength is related to the proper laying down of collagen), aloe reverses this problem, whether taken orally or applied locally to the wound.[18] If the same holds true for humans, that means glyconutrients lessen the chance of a wound reopening—still another reason to consider applying aloe to cuts and burns.

To remove acne scars and wrinkles, dermatologists and plastic surgeons use facial dermabrasion, in which the outer layers of skin are sanded down with a stainless steel brush or diamond-fraise wheel. Afterward, the patient's face oozes blood and serum; scabs last a few weeks. In one case study, directly following the dermabrasion procedure and for five days after, one side of a patient's face was treated with standard wound dressing, while the other side was treated with standard wound dressing and stabilized *Aloe vera* gel.[19] Forty-eight hours later researchers found that the aloe-treated side was less swollen and inflamed than the control side. By the fourth day there was less oozing and crusting on the aloe side, and by the sixth day healing on the aloe side was complete—three days faster than the control side.

*Suggested Use for Small Wounds and Cuts:* For large and serious wounds, see a physician immediately. (You may need stitches, antibiotics, or a tetanus shot.) For small cuts, after cleansing the wound, break open a leaf from an *Aloe vera* plant and use the clear inner gel to coat the affected area, or use stabilized gel on the wound several times a day. Cover the wound with gauze if you're going out; otherwise leave uncovered.

*Suggested Use for Dermatological Surgery:* Talk to your doctor if you are thinking about taking glyconutrients before or after a surgical procedure, including dermabrasion, to safeguard against possible allergic reactions. Some glyconutrients, including reishi, cordyceps, and pectins, can increase bleeding and should *not* be used a week before or in the week following surgery.

Whenever applying *Aloe vera* for the first time, dab on a little in an inconspicuous spot on your leg or arm and wait twenty-four hours to see if you develop an allergic reaction. If skin becomes red and itchy or you develop hives, discontinue use.

## Chapter 9

# Addressing Chronic Fatigue Syndrome, Fibromyalgia, and Gulf War Syndrome

*These debilitating illnesses often respond to glyconutrient supplementation.*

The causes of chronic fatigue syndrome, fibromyalgia, and Gulf War syndrome have not been fully explained, but the consequence is immune dysfunction. Glyconutrients help the body fight off bacterial, fungal, parasitic, and viral infections (particularly herpes), which often accompany these diseases. Glyconutrients also generate antioxidants and improve the functioning of the key immune cells, including macrophages and natural killer cells, which tend to be depressed in these illnesses. In addition, several studies indicate that glyconutrients increase endurance in both animals and humans; it stands to reason that glyconutrients may boost stamina in patients with these energy-depleting illnesses.[1, 2] (For more information on saccharides' ability to bolster stamina, see chapter 13.)

Glyconutrients can be helpful in mitigating symptoms in these diseases by protecting the brain from the effects of histamine and toxins: people with these disorders tend to be allergic and release too much histamine (for more information on histamine, see chapter 7), and they tend to be sensitive to environmental toxins; indeed, some patients can point to a toxic exposure as the trigger for their illness.

Chronic fatigue syndrome (CFS) is known by many names. In the United States it's also called chronic fatigue immune dysfunction syndrome, or CFIDS; in England it's termed myalgic encephalomyelitis, or ME for short; and in Japan it's sometimes called low natural killer cell disease because the number of natural killer cells is often low and those present often function poorly.[3]

Fatigue—the kind of fatigue that renders you too exhausted to lift a hairbrush or walk to the mailbox—is just the tip of the iceberg in CFS, which is also marked by mental confusion, short-term memory problems, and autonomic nervous system abnormalities. (Standing and even sitting often result in blood pressure falling precipitously.) About 10 percent of people with the disorder experience seizures, and, curiously, some patients lose their fingerprints. Most disquieting for many with the disorder are the cognitive difficulties. While verbal IQ is usually spared, visual and spatial right-brain functions can be hit hard.

CFS patients often lose the ability to find their way home from familiar places; lose the ability to do simple math, particularly subtraction; and misplace familiar items in bizarre places. As investigative reporter Hillary Johnson explains in her book *Osler's Web: Inside the Labyrinth of the Chronic Fatigue Syndrome Epidemic*, one frustrated patient, a lawyer, told his doctor he was upset because he had misplaced his wallet. When the doctor tried to calm down the man, with the usual bromide that everyone misplaces things on occasion, the patient shot back, "You don't understand. When I found my wallet, it was in the freezer compartment of the refrigerator."[4] Another patient, writes Johnson, informed her doctor that she had tried to make a pay phone call by slipping a quarter into a parking meter.[5]

Patients describe CFS as feeling as if you have Alzheimer's disease, lupus, arthritis, multiple sclerosis, and the flu all wrapped up into one—and you've just run a marathon. And it's no wonder:

The constellation of symptoms includes low-grade fevers and chills, lymph node enlargement, sore throats, night sweats, painful joints and muscles, and sleep disorders. Many also suffer from chronic yeast, bladder, and upper respiratory infections; allergies; and food and drug sensitivities.

Gulf War syndrome mimics the symptoms of CFS—in fact, some researchers believe the two illnesses are one and the same. In both syndromes, an identical piece of chromosome 22 often exhibits a curious, acquired abnormality,[6] possibly induced by a virus, bacterium, vaccine, or toxin. Veterans with Gulf War syndrome, like CFS patients, exhibit poor natural killer cell function.[7] Afflicting an estimated 100,000 men and women who served during the Gulf War, the malady was deemed erroneously to be a posttraumatic stress disorder by many experts until recently. These days, the effects of multiple vaccines as well as chemical and biological warfare on the Desert Storm veterans are being considered as potential causes or contributors.

Fibromyalgia presents in patients with trigger points in the muscles that hurt acutely to the touch. One of my acquaintances with the disorder feels exquisite pain during her worst moments just from the scanty weight of the clothes on her body. Sleep disorders and irritable bowel syndrome are also common. And many people with fibromyalgia exhibit CFS symptoms, including poor natural killer cell function,[8] just as those with CFS often demonstrate the tender points of fibromyalgia.

Not long ago, physicians wrote off these enigmatic diseases as inconsequential or psychosomatic because patients' physical exams were often unremarkable, and there was no straightforward test to establish the diagnosis. Today, there still is no straightforward test, but that dismissive view is finally changing. Years of published research conducted at Harvard, Vanderbilt, Johns Hopkins, and the University of Pennsylvania point to immune dysfunction and cardiac abnormalities in these illnesses.

Some medical experts, however, continue to trumpet their disbelief in these diseases as if they were illusions in the minds of the afflicted. Doctors who don't believe in the reality of CFS, fibromyalgia, and Gulf War syndrome usually diagnose these patients with depression. But, in fact, people with clinical depression usually register high levels of cortisol—a steroid produced by the adrenal gland—while those with CFS generally have low levels.[9] In addition, in clinical depression, both verbal and nonverbal IQs usually drop. In CFS and Gulf War syndrome, however, researchers have found what's called "intellectual scatter": certain functions of the brain hum along normally while others may be severely impaired.[10] This kind of focal brain dysfunction is seen in people who have organic brain disease or have suffered strokes—it's not the pattern seen in clinical depression.

Sadly, however, the psychiatric bias against these physical diseases persists. In the history of medicine, psychological causes are often ascribed to otherwise unexplained diseases until the real agent is found. Such was the case many years ago with multiple sclerosis, epilepsy, and, more recently, AIDS. In fact, at the turn of the twentieth century, medical journals dubbed multiple sclerosis the "faker's disease," and one physician-endorsed treatment for epilepsy was a sound beating. Nearly eighty years later, gay men in San Francisco with swollen lymph nodes and night sweats were shrugged off by their doctors as the worried well, as writer Randy Shilts documented eloquently in the book *And the Band Played On.*[11]

## Treating Immune Dysfunction

Studies on people with CFS show that when their natural killer cells and other key immune cells aren't fully functional, an accelerated form of programmed cell death occurs, and the immune cells can't kill invading organisms with their normal power.[12, 13] What's encouraging is that animal and in vitro studies indicate that glyconutrients (including maitake, cordyceps, and reishi mushrooms, as well as rice bran, arabinogalactans, and polysaccharide K), have been shown to enhance natural killer cell capability.[14, 15, 16, 17, 18]

Lentinan, an extract of the shiitake mushroom, has been tested in a double-blind trial in CFS patients in Japan, where the

disease is prevalent. Researchers found that all twenty-three patients ages fourteen to seventy-seven who received an intramus-
cular injection or intravenous infusion (over the course of one
hour) of 1 gram of lentinan every other day or twice a week experienced a return to normal natural killer activity.[19] Curiously,
however, during treatment natural killer activity at first *declined* in
the participants, a peculiar lentinan effect that's been observed
in cancer patients but not in healthy people taking the glyconutrient. With continued administration of lentinan for six months,
however, natural killer activity returned to the normal range. In
addition, the glyconutrient activated killer T cells and interferon. These immune system agents also function abnormally in
CFS as well as in Gulf War syndrome and fibromyalgia.[20]

*Suggested Use:* Oral lentinan is sold as a food supplement; the
recommended dose is 12.5 milligrams once or twice a day. While
generally less effective than injectable lentinan, the oral form
has shown efficacy in treating other viruses, including venereal
warts (see chapter 5).

Injectable and intravenous lentinan are available by prescription and must be administered only under physician supervision.
Serious side effects have occurred, and they include fever, chills,
back and leg pain, elevated liver enzymes, and anaphylaxis—a
serious and potentially fatal allergic reaction. Doses are calculated by a physician according to the patient's weight and health
status. (See the resources chapter for more information.) Dietary supplementation with other glyconutrients and mushrooms should also be considered—starting at low doses and
increasing gradually over a month.

## Preventing Infections

Immune dysfunction sometimes results in more frequent infections in patients with CFS, fibromyalgia, and Gulf War syndrome,
but in animal trials, saccharides curb bacterial infections from
*E. coli* and strep and help protect the body from viruses, including the flu.[21, 22, 23] Glyconutrients, particularly polysaccharide K

and acemannan from aloe, also help the body fight off the yeast infections that are common in these illnesses.[24, 25]

*Suggested Use:* Until human trials are conducted, we won't know if glyconutrients will curb infections from *E. coli*, yeast, and other microbes in people. Nevertheless, supporting the body with any of the glyconutrients listed in the Suggested Use sections in this chapter may help improve immune functioning in CFS, fibromyalgia, and Gulf War syndrome. Follow the manufacturer's recommendations or your doctor's advice.

## Boosting Antioxidant Activity

Antioxidants, particularly glutathione, are in short supply in CFS, fibromyalgia, and Gulf War syndrome; an increase in free-radical generation often occurs as well.[26] In human studies, cordyceps extracts and Cs-4 have been shown to scavenge free radicals and so may be beneficial.[27] And in animal and in vitro studies, *Aloe vera* extracts, polysaccharide K, and reishi mushrooms have been potent stimulators of glutathione, which destroys free radicals.[28, 29, 30]

*Suggested Use:* Cordyceps extract or Cs-4: 1 to 6 grams a day, in divided doses to help promote free-radical scavenging. Do not take cordyceps or Cs-4 if you have a bleeding disorder or are taking a blood-thinner unless you have your doctor's approval. Though oral glutathione is not well absorbed, some patients report that supplementing with the amino acid is helpful—though others have found that it exacerbates their symptoms. Consult with your doctor before trying glutathione and follow his or her dosing recommendations.

## Viral Causes of Immune-Deficient Diseases

Some scientists believe a single agent is responsible for CFS, fibromyalgia, and Gulf War syndrome. Others think the causes are multifactorial: Various viruses, retroviruses, bacteria, fungi, spirochetes, vaccines, and toxins, along with genetic susceptibility, have been implicated as working together. Hepatitis C has been linked to some cases of fibromyalgia (particularly in young women), and back in the 1980s, the Epstein-Barr virus—the herpes virus that sets off mononucleosis—was deemed the architect of CFS. This theory has since been debunked, though the Epstein-Barr virus is often reactivated in the disorder, as are other herpes viruses.*

Whatever the exact role herpes viruses play in immune-deficient diseases, anecdotal evidence and in vitro studies indicate that glyconutrients are effective against these viruses.[31, 32, 33] By increasing the activity of the natural killer cells, polysaccharide K, for instance, has efficacy against cytomegalovirus, a herpes virus that can wreak havoc on the immunocompromised.[34] We also know that in animals and humans, herpes I and II viruses infect by attaching to specific glycoproteins on the skin or mucous membranes of the mouth or genitalia.[35] Glyconutrients suppress herpes viruses, causing them to produce abnormal or uninfectious glycoproteins rather than by killing the viruses directly.[36, 37]

Recently, scientists have zeroed in on another herpes virus, human herpes virus 6 (HHV-6), commonly found in DNA extracted from the blood cells of people with Gulf War syndrome and CFS.[38] Most of us have been exposed to the virus at some point in our lives, but it goes dormant if the body's immune system is functioning optimally. As discussed in Nicholas Regush's book *The Virus Within*, researchers Konnie Knox and Donald Carrigan have reported that the virus is active in up to 70 percent of those with CFS that they have tested—though whether the pathogen is the cause, co-factor, or just part of the cascade effect of a damaged immune system has not been determined.[39] Other researchers are also reporting an HHV-6 connection, finding a significant elevation of antibody as well as active HHV-6 infection in CFS patients, compared with controls.[40]

---

*Some physicians still mislabel CFS as chronic Epstein-Barr, sometimes out of ignorance but more often to spare their patients the discomfiture that the trivializing label chronic fatigue syndrome bestows. With the hectic lives we lead, who, after all, doesn't get tired?

Whether glyconutrients work on HHV-6 is unknown, but as they're effective on other herpes viruses, and as glyconutrients boost general immunity, it may be worth a shot to try them. (For more information on herpes viruses and glyconutrients, see chapter 5.)

*Suggested Use:* I recommend several glyconutrients, individually or together, to treat viral manifestations of these illnesses. If you are allergic to mushrooms, do not take cordyceps extracts or Cs-4. Otherwise, with your doctor's approval, try cordyceps extracts or Cs-4: 1 to 3 grams a day, in divided doses. If you have a bleeding disorder or take blood thinners, do not use cordyceps extracts without your doctor's okay. Your blood thinners might need to be adjusted or discontinued by your doctor if you are a good candidate for the extract.

Aloe extracts: 250 milligrams once or twice a day. Arabinogalactans: 1 to 1.5 grams daily, in divided doses. AHCC: 1 to 3 grams in divided doses. Caution: People with CFS, fibromyalgia, and Gulf War syndrome are often acutely sensitive to foods, vitamins, and medications, and should start slowly with one glyconutrient at a time and build up gradually. If you combine two glyconutrients, cut the dose for each by half; if you combine three, cut the dose for each by two-thirds, and so on. Consider adding cooked shiitake, maitake, and oyster mushrooms to your diet.

## Mycoplasmas

While virus research takes center stage in CFS, fibromyalgia, and Gulf War syndrome, some scientists are investigating antibiotic-sensitive microbes. A scientist at Vanderbilt University suggests that the organism responsible for CFS and fibromyalgia, as well as multiple sclerosis, is *Chlamydia pneumoniae.*[41] It's a mycoplasma— a kind of a cross between a bacteria and a virus that responds to antibiotics. The organism has also been implicated in heart disease. But other researchers believe another mycoplasma is the culprit in Gulf War syndrome and CFS: *Mycoplasma pneumo-*

*niae.*[42, 43] AIDS patients often come down with the infection as well.

*Suggested Use:* If you have a mycoplasma infection, you must see your doctor. Saccharide studies on mycoplasmas have yet to be conducted, but supplementing with glyconutrient-rich foods or supplements can help bolster your overall immunity. Follow the manufacturer's directions or your doctor's advice.

## Parasites

The latest theory to emerge about the causes of CFS is that a newly discovered parasite, christened *Cryptostrongylus pulmoni* (hidden lungworm) by its discoverer Dr. Larry Klapow, is a contributor. This roundworm, postulates Klapow, made its way to Southeast Asia from its native Australia, and was brought to the United States during the Vietnam War.[44] The worm can contaminate food and water—as well as the blood of its animal and human hosts. Most other worms can be detected with a stool test, but *Cryptostrongylus* purportedly travels clandestinely for years from its victims' lungs to intestines—and back again—navigating through blood vessels and gut walls, wreaking havoc without detection. Until scientists devise a blood test, the only way to recover the worm is by examining sputum produced by a deep cough, a painstaking procedure with many false negatives.

Studies indicate that glyconutrients are effective against parasites, but it's not known if glyconutrients equip the body to challenge *C. pulmoni.*[45, 46] (See chapter 6 for more information on glyconutrients' effects on parasites.)

*Suggested Use:* If you believe you may have a parasitic infection, see your doctor. Although effective drugs are available to treat parasites, it's not known if they will kill *C. pulmoni.* Nor is it known whether glyconutrients are effective against *C. pulmoni.* Beta-glucans from mushrooms, yeast, oat, barley, and rice have been shown to be effective against certain parasites in animal and test-tube studies—but that's a long way from human trials. To improve general immune functioning, consider supplementing with cooked maitake, shiitake, and oyster mushrooms to bring beta-glucan polysaccharides into your diet.

## Cytokine Activity

While some cell functions stall in CFS, Gulf War syndrome, and fibromyalgia, others rev up into overdrive—and in this way these ailments mimic autoimmune diseases. Levels of cytokines— proteins activated in the immune system response—register as high or higher in people with CFS, fibromyalgia, and Gulf War syndrome as in those with allergies.[47, 48, 49] The high levels of these cytokines combined with the reactivation of latent viruses suggest to some experts that the body is trying, albeit unsuccessfully, to shake off some kind of pathogen, be it a bacterium, a virus, or a parasite. To operate effectively cytokines must interface with properly formed cell-surface glycoprotein receptors. But the receptors are often defective in these diseases. For instance, scientists have found that CFS patients show a drop in cell glycoproteins that are critical to launching a proper immune response.[50] And the sicker the patient, the more severe the glycoprotein abnormalities tend to be.

When these glycoproteins are defective, the cells are likely to produce larger quantities of cytokines to overcome the dysfunction. Think about it this way: Suppose you try to wake somebody from sleep. You call her name. No response. You open the curtains. Still nothing. You shake her. Nada. You scream her name and slam the door. Now this is becoming scary. Just as you might shout to try to rouse someone in deep sleep, the body "shouts" in its own way, by ratcheting up its stimulus (cytokines) until it gets a sufficient response from its lethargic, insensitive immune system that's oblivious to an invading virus, toxin, or bacterium. The body gets thrown into a state of panic because the immune system is not heeding its wake-up calls.

So how do you turn on the switch and get the body to heed the cytokine wake-up calls? In CFS, fibromyalgia, and Gulf War syndrome, some researchers believe the body tends toward what's called a Th2 or humoral response, in which B cells produce antibodies that float in the blood and neutralize or destroy unwanted particles or organisms. There is convincing evidence that many people with CFS, fibromyalgia, or Gulf War syndrome had allergies long before they got sick—and allergies are evidence of this overaggressive humoral response.[51] And as discussed earlier, people with CFS often register high antibody levels to herpes viruses, among other viruses, which again indicates a Th2 response. Even though the formation of antibodies is crucial in the immune-system cascade—they're why vaccines work, for instance—antibodies are only half of the story.

The other half is a strong cell-mediated response called Th1, which is needed to fight such diseases as typhoid and tuberculosis and perhaps CFS, fibromyalgia, and Gulf War syndrome as well. In Th1, the body launches immune cells that directly annihilate pathogens, and certain cytokines predominate. Perhaps shifting the balance from a Th2 to Th1 response is what's needed in CFS, fibromyalgia, and Gulf War syndrome. This doesn't mean that Th2 is "bad" and Th1 is "good." Either kind of immune pathway activated inappropriately or excessively could be a source of problems.

One of the theories postulated by researchers at the University College of London Medical School is that multiple vaccinations of the Gulf War troops caused a systemic shift toward a Th2 response.[52] It's possible that calming down the antibody response and activating the cellular response may effect healing.

This is where glyconutrients come in: they enable the body to immunomodulate—to arrest the immune system where and when it's overreacting as well as to boost immune-system components that aren't responding in full force.[53] In a Vanderbilt University study, for instance, when cytotoxic T cells—which kill invaders directly as part of the Th1-mediated immunity—were fed acemannan from aloe, both their number and their capacity to destroy a challenge increased.[54]

*Suggested Use:* We don't know conclusively that saccharides can shift the body from a Th2 to a Th1 response in patients with CFS, fibromyalgia, and Gulf War syndrome—or even if that's what needs to be done. But again, taking any of the glyconutrients listed under Suggested Use in this chapter may improve immune functioning.

## Treating Cognitive Function

CFS and Gulf War syndrome patients often experience short-term memory problems; some fibromyalgia patients do as well. German researchers have found that in test-tube studies saccharides can improve memory formation.[55] In addition, many patients with these disorders are sensitive to drugs and environmental allergens as well as to foods (particularly wheat, caffeinated coffee, and chocolate) and additives (NutraSweet and MSG are major culprits). Their allergic responses to sundry substances lead to an overproduction of histamine and contribute to what patients term "brain fog." Glyconutrients can help: reishi extracts have been found to inhibit histamine release and curb allergic reactions in rodents.[56]

Alcohol is particularly problematic for patients with these disorders. For many, even a glass of wine can bring on symptoms in spades. But in several animal studies, glyconutrients have been shown to protect the brain from alcohol's intoxicating effects.[57, 58, 59, 60] Perhaps if saccharides can shield the overtaxed brain from such toxic assaults as alcohol, these sugars may also safeguard the brain from other assaults, including those from viruses and bacteria, enabling brain functioning to improve.

*Suggested Use:* Because the reishi studies on histamine release and the glyconutrient studies on preventing alcohol intoxication have been conducted only on animals, we don't know if the effects apply to humans. But supplementing with reishi extracts and other glyconutrients can strengthen the immune system. Reishi extracts: 1 to 6 grams daily, in divided doses. Do not take reishi extracts if you are on a blood thinner or have a bleeding disorder unless under a doctor's care.

## Blood Hypercoagulability

Scientists in Arizona have recently discovered that some CFS and fibromyalgia patients have blood hypercoagulability, caused by an overproduction of fibrin, which makes the blood clot too easily. This can potentially lead to heart attacks and strokes unless patients are treated with blood thinners like heparin.[61] In particular, the researchers have found that one unusual blood marker called LP(a) is often elevated in CFS. Tennis great Arthur Ashe, who had an abnormally high LP(a) level, suffered a heart attack at the age of thirty-seven. Along with prescription blood thinners, mushrooms may be helpful here: cordyceps and reishi mushrooms contain adenosine, a nucleotide that is a structural unit of our DNA. Adenosine's blood-thinning effects have been shown to reduce the formation of clots in rabbits.[62] Pectins have blood-thinning effects as well.[63]

*Suggested Use:* Do not use pectins or cordyceps or reishi extracts if you have a bleeding disorder unless under a doctor's care. Consult your doctor before trying glyconutrients to reduce fibrin levels, particularly if you are already on blood-thinning medication, such as heparin, Plavix, aspirin, NSAIDS like ibuprofen, and Cox-2 inhibitors like Vioxx. You need to be monitored closely because thinning the blood too much can cause bleeding. If and only if your doctor gives you the go-ahead, try *one* of the following glyconutrients: pectins, 5 grams, two to three times a day; reishi extract, 3 to 6 grams a day, in divided doses; cordyceps extracts or Cs-4, 3 to 6 grams a day, in divided doses. Caution: Some patients with these illnesses taking drugs to thin the blood report a *worsening* of symptoms. If your symptoms worsen on glyconutrients, discontinue the glyconutrients and consult your physician.

## Chronic Diseases

Fibromyalgia is a chronic condition, but the conventional wisdom has been that most people eventually recovered from Gulf

War syndrome and CFS. In reality, however, after the first two years the odds of recovery for all three illnesses grow slim. In one study conducted in the Netherlands, for instance, only 3 percent of 246 CFS patients reported complete recovery after eighteen months with the disease, with another 17 percent reporting improvement.[64] After a while many patients admit they've forgotten what it feels like to be well, making it difficult to gauge how they do feel. "If it weren't for the fact that I can't do anything, I would think that I had recovered," one longtime CFS sufferer told her doctor, Paul Cheney, who began treating the disease in the mid-1980s, during an outbreak in the posh resort town of Incline Village, Nevada.

At present there is no cure for CFS, fibromyalgia, or Gulf War syndrome. Instead, physicians treat the symptoms, prescribing agents for sleep, pain, and low blood pressure. Unfortunately, drug companies aren't doing much research, in part because many researchers continue to insist that the illnesses are psychiatric. And according to the Associated Press and the *Washington Post*, a government audit turned up the finding that at least 8.8 million CFS research dollars—that's 39 percent of the funds earmarked for CFS research over several years—was funneled off by the Centers for Disease Control in Atlanta for research on measles and polio, among other diseases.[65, 66]

Although glyconutrients may not be a cure for CFS, fibromyalgia, or Gulf War syndrome, they can help strengthen an overtaxed, battle-weary immune system. For many that will bring a mitigation of symptoms. For some people, particularly if their illnesses are caught early, saccharides may enable their immune systems to turn the corner and get on the mend.

## Chapter 10

# Managing Arthritis, Diabetes, and Other Chronic Illnesses

---

*The beneficial effects of glyconutrients on arthritis, diabetes, Crohn's disease, ulcerative colitis, interstitial cystitis, lupus, kidney disease, and transplants.*

### OSTEOARTHRITIS: A PATIENT'S SUCCESS

Christie is a fifty-three-year-old social worker with a type of arthritis in her knees and back called osteoarthritis, in which the cartilage that cushions the joints degenerates, causing pain, stiffness, and swelling. In the past few years her condition had worsened considerably. Her pain slowed down her mobility, which in turn caused her to gain 10 pounds, adding more weight to her already-stressed joints. For the pain, she often donned knee braces and took Tylenol or ibuprofen four to five times a week. On one occasion last year her knee swelled more than usual, and the excruciating pain was unremitting; her doctor withdrew some fluid from her knee with a needle and then injected steroids to reduce the inflammation.

After seeing a segment on the news about the benefits of glucosamine—a metabolic product of the essential saccharide

N-acetylglucosamine—and chondroitin, a polysaccharide found in cartilage, Christie decided the supplements were worth a try. She picked up a bottle of each at her health food store and added 1,500 milligrams of glucosamine and 1,200 milligrams of chondroitin to her regimen, as per the manufacturer's recommendations. Within a couple of months, her pain and stiffness had eased considerably, and she cut back on her pain meds to about once a week.

## Osteoarthritis

Cartilage is a smooth white material that's coated with a slippery lubricating liquid called synovial fluid. Healthy joints, crowned with cartilage and bathed in synovial fluid, move smoothly, silently, and effortlessly, with the cartilage serving as a shock absorber, especially in the knees and the hips, which bear the brunt of our weight. Cartilage is composed of glycoproteins called collagen and proteoglycans. When the wear and tear on cartilage exceeds the ability of the body to generate new cartilage, osteoarthritis occurs. In the United States alone, more than 16 million people have the disease, which is particularly common in people over sixty, though the symptoms may be mild. Nonsteroidal anti-inflammatories like Motrin and Naprosyn provide symptom relief, but they don't address the root problem and can cause stomach bleeding and toxicity to the kidneys. And, ironically, their chronic use may worsen the course of the disease by enhancing the production of inflammatory mediators called cytokines and inhibiting cartilage repair.[1]

Glucosamine does more than relieve symptoms: it helps repair damage. The glyconutrient has become a popular remedy for osteoarthritis, but there's science behind the claims. Studies show that glucosamine encourages cartilage rebuilding, increases range of motion, and decreases pain in the disease.[2, 3] In fact, results of a placebo-controlled study of 212 patients with osteoarthritis published in 2001 in the British journal *Lancet* found that, unlike the dummy drug, 1,500 milligrams of glucosamine sulfate daily for three years alleviated arthritis symptoms, prevented further damage, and repaired some of the existing damage by rebuilding cartilage. Belgian, British, Italian, and American researchers collaborated on the three-year trial; all the patients had osteoarthritis of the knee, a prime spot for the disease.

And in another, recent, controlled study, orthopedists in Israel found that patients with osteoarthritis of the knee who were given intravenous glucosamine and 800 milligrams daily of oral chondroitin for four weeks showed significant improvement in range of motion and relief from knee pain and tenderness, as compared with controls, who showed no improvement.[4] The researchers concluded that these glyconutrients were safe and effective for prolonged treatment of osteoarthritis.

Jane Brody, health columnist for the *New York Times*, suffers from osteoarthritis in her knees and has written about her success using glucosamine and chondroitin to treat her condition. After her eleven-year-old arthritic spaniel improved dramatically on the supplement combination, she decided to give the supplements a go. Two months later she reported a 30 percent improvement. "I am not pain-free," she wrote, "and I still tend to get a little stiff after prolonged sitting, but I have stopped limping, I am playing tennis and ice skating with less pain and my knees have stopped swelling after strenuous activity."[5] She takes a brand manufactured by Nutramax Laboratories called Cosamin (her dog takes the animal version, Cosequin). Each capsule supplies 500 milligrams of glucosamine and 400 milligrams of chondroitin, plus small amounts of vitamin C and manganese to enhance absorption; Brody takes three capsules daily. (See the resources section for more information.)

*Suggested Use:* 1,500 milligrams of glucosamine and 1,200 milligrams of chondroitin daily, in three divided doses. Rarely, glucosamine and chondroitin cause stomach discomfort; if this occurs, take the glyconutrients with food, cut down your intake, or discontinue.

## Autoimmune Illnesses

Osteoarthritis is a degenerative form of arthritis, whereas rheumatoid arthritis is an autoimmune form of the disease. When treating autoimmune disease, I was taught as a medical student, "When in doubt . . . use steroids!" Sadly, steroids are still the mainstay. Long-term patients with rheumatoid arthritis, lupus, ulcerative colitis, and other autoimmune disorders are often resigned to steroids, though some eventually press their doctors for alternatives. Unfortunately, the only available alternatives are problematic drugs such as the toxic cancer medications methotrexate and cyclophosphamide.

Western medicine is poorly equipped to treat these diseases. Steroids abruptly halt the immune system's function when it appears as if its actions are going to cause damage. These drugs are undeniably useful for short-term problems—in severe allergic reactions, for instance, steroids can bring about a speedy and full recovery. But over the long term, patients often pay a high price because steroids can also cause severe damage to the tissues, bones, health, and immunity.

There are exceptions, of course. People with Addison's disease take a steroid replacement dose daily because the adrenal gland, which normally manufactures these hormones, stops functioning partially or entirely, leading to kidney shutdown and death. In many cases, however, the disease processes for which steroids are used aren't resolved with treatment—they're just frozen in time until the steroids are withdrawn, which often leads to a flare-up or a worsening of the disease, which leads to more steroids, and the vicious cycle continues, with higher and higher doses. "When the steroids stop working," confided a friend with lupus, "and you've gained 30 pounds and your bones are getting brittle and your face grows round as the moon, they'll put you on a nasty cocktail of cancer drugs. And you'll yearn for those good old days when you first went on steroids." Unfortunately, the alternative for someone in a lupus crisis—when, for instance, the kidneys shut down—may be death. So steroids seem the lesser of the two evils, the best we have. Or are they?

In human and animal studies, glyconutrients have been shown to improve blood-work results and quiet autoimmune symptoms—reversing poor kidney function caused by longstanding lupus (see the Lupus and Kidney Disease sections of this chapter for more information), relieving inflammation from rheumatoid arthritis (see the Rheumatoid Arthritis section for more), stabilizing blood sugar in juvenile diabetics (see the Diabetes sections), and healing unsightly plaques from psoriasis (see chapter 8). One of the reasons glyconutrients may work is that saccharide formation is disturbed in these illnesses.

Compared with healthy controls, for instance, patients with rheumatoid arthritis, Crohn's disease, juvenile-onset arthritis, and Sjögren's syndrome (characterized by dry, irritated mucous membranes) register disturbances in the essential saccharides galactose and N-acetylglucosamine.[6] Researchers believe that the abnormal readings result from errors in glycosylation, which occur when saccharides are added to proteins to form more complex structures. And the result of these glycosylation errors is that the immune system receives faulty messages that mark certain cells as foreign: autoimmune disease results when the immune system attacks cells that it's supposed to protect. Adding saccharides to the diet may—theoretically at least—help mitigate autoimmune symptoms by correcting abnormal glycosylation.

## Rheumatoid Arthritis

A deficiency in galactose, another essential saccharide, has been implicated in rheumatoid arthritis, which causes joint stiffness, inflammation, and sometimes deformity. Interestingly, small studies, including one at Leipzig University in Germany, indicate that of fifty participants with early rheumatoid arthritis of no more than two years in duration, about 70 percent registered a galactose deficiency, compared with about 10 percent of normal controls.[7] In fact, galactose shortage was a better indicator of arthritis than a positive rheumatoid factor, a standard blood marker for arthritis. But whether supplementing the diet with galactose will help mitigate disease symptoms hasn't been determined. Galactose is plentiful in milk and milk products, so most people get enough of this saccharide naturally. For people with lactose intolerance, who get diarrhea and cramping from eating dairy, there are alternatives. Figs, grapes, peas (particularly black-eyed peas), tomatoes, hazelnuts, and many kinds of beans, including garbanzo, navy, and kidney, are rich in galactose. Pectin supplements also contain galactose.

We know more about aloe's effects on arthritis, at least in animals. When researchers treated arthritic rats with *Aloe vera*, the result was a 50 percent decrease in inflammation.[8] Mast cells, activated in allergic and autoimmune phenomena, also decreased, by 48 percent. In addition, the aloe stimulated an increase in fibroblasts, which grow and repair the tissue. Other studies indicate that aloe extracts markedly inhibit induced arthritis, edema, and inflammation in rodents.[9, 10]

*Suggested Use:* Unfortunately, no human trials have been done to determine aloe's effects on rheumatoid arthritis in humans, so I can't yet recommend the glyconutrient to treat the illness. For improving general immune function, supplementing with standardized, powdered *Aloe vera* extract can be helpful, 500 milligrams to 1 gram a day, in divided doses.

## Diabetes

Diabetes results either when the body isn't making enough insulin, a hormone produced by the pancreas to regulate blood sugar, or when the body is insensitive to the insulin being generated. In type I, or juvenile diabetes, the body produces little or no insulin because the pancreatic cells that normally create it have been destroyed, usually by an autoimmune phenomenon that may occur after a viral infection, when antibodies and immune cells are raised against the cells of the pancreas. People with type I diabetes must take insulin.

Type II, or adult-onset diabetes, is not an autoimmune disease. Although the symptoms are similar to those of juvenile diabetes, they may be less pronounced and usually occur later in
life. People with adult-onset diabetes can often manage their disease with diet and pills; some require insulin, particularly as the
diseases progresses. Adult-onset diabetes occurs more commonly
in overweight individuals older than forty, though we are beginning to see type II diabetes in overweight, sedentary children
and adolescents. In this subgroup, the problem is not a lack of
insulin, at least initially. If anything, people in this group produce too much insulin, but they appear to respond poorly to it—
they're insulin resistant, so the body has to produce more and
more of the hormone to regulate blood sugar.

Why this happens isn't clear, but it's been theorized that the
insulin receptors, which are glycoproteins, are faulty. Foods like
white rice, pasta, bread, and processed, sucrose-laden snacks with
a high glycemic index—a measure of the speed at which glucose
enters the bloodstream—exacerbate the problem. These foods
increase the blood-sugar level, and in response, the body produces more insulin to bring it down. Over time, high insulin levels damage blood vessels and increase the levels of low-density
lipoprotein (LDL), the so-called bad cholesterol. The sugars in
glyconutrients don't cause insulin problems for diabetics because the amounts in an average daily supplement are very small,
and glucose is just one of the eight essential saccharides: the
other saccharides have lower glycemic indexes.

## Adult-Onset, Type II Diabetes

*Aloe vera* is effective at lowering blood glucose in type II diabetes.
In a very small study of five patients with noninsulin-dependent
diabetes, half a teaspoon of stabilized *Aloe vera* powder daily for
four to fourteen weeks resulted in a significant drop in blood
sugar from a mean of 273 to 151 (70 to 110 is normal) with no
change in body weight.[11]

In another, larger study of 72 patients aged thirty-five to seventy years with adult-onset diabetes, researchers found that 1 tablespoon of *Aloe vera* juice, in combination with the oral diabetes drug glibenclamide, was effective in lowering blood glucose and triglycerides.[12] Researchers at Mahidol University in Bangkok gave the treatment group aloe juice plus glibenclamide, while the control group received a placebo juice plus glibenclamide. After forty-two days, levels of fasting blood glucose and triglycerides of the aloe-treated group—but not the controls—were lowered significantly (see Table 2). Cholesterol changes weren't significant in either group. The researchers also monitored liver and kidney function during the course of the trial and found no toxicity problems from *Aloe vera*.

TABLE 2. ALOE VERA PLUS GLIBENCLAMIDE VERSUS GLIBENCLAMIDE PLUS PLACEBO IN TREATING ADULT-ONSET, TYPE II DIABETES

|  | Control (Placebo and Glibenclamide) | Treated (Aloe Vera and Glibenclamide) |
|---|---|---|
| BLOOD SUGAR LEVELS | | |
| Day 1 | 289 | 288 |
| Day 14 | 279 | 231 |
| Day 42 | 289 | 148 |
| BLOOD CHOLESTEROL | | |
| Day 1 | 235 | 229 |
| Day 14 | 237 | 227 |
| Day 42 | 243 | 225 |
| BLOOD TRIGLYCERIDES | | |
| Day 1 | 222 | 264 |
| Day 14 | 222 | 219 |
| Day 42 | 233 | 128 |

## ADULT-ONSET, TYPE II DIABETES:
## A PATIENT'S SUCCESS

Sid is a seventy-six-year-old retired postal worker who's had adult-onset diabetes for twenty-one years. He's thirty pounds overweight; obesity is a risk factor for adult-onset diabetes and losing even a few pounds can result in tremendous benefit. Five years ago, Sid's doctor started him on insulin because his diabetic pills and diet were not controlling his diabetes. Six months ago, in a move to improve his overall health, Sid also started taking glyconutrients: 250 milligrams of yeast beta-glucans and 500 milligrams of powdered aloe extracts daily. Within a week, he started suffering hypoglycemic attacks, which occur when blood sugar drops too low. His symptoms included tingling of the fingers, intense hunger, and faintness. It seemed his cells had become more responsive to insulin, and suddenly the dosage of insulin his doctor had prescribed was too much. His doctor reduced the dose, and within a month Sid was weaned off insulin altogether. Buoyed by the improvement in his health—no more needles!—Sid has begun exercising, taking a brisk walk every day, and the pounds are starting to come off.

In animals, studies indicate that glyconutrients lower plasma glucose, plasma insulin, and urinary glucose and reduce food intake in genetically diabetic mice.[13, 14, 15]

Maitake mushrooms are effective in diabetic mice called KK-A$^y$. These mice have a double-whammy: they have diabetes and obesity, and both problems get worse with age. Japanese researchers placed one group of these mice on a maitake-enhanced feed from pulverized, dehydrated maitake mushrooms; the controls received standard feed.[16] After eight weeks, the glucose level of the maitake group remained stable at 200, compared with 400 for controls. In addition, blood insulin and triglyceride levels doubled in the controls, unlike the maitake group, which remained stable on both counts. What's more, after eight weeks, the maitake rats were thinner, averaging 10 grams less than the controls.

Not all glyconutrient studies in diabetes—at least in animals—have been promising, however. In particular, a 1994 study on diabetic rats showed that *Aloe vera* gel given orally twice daily for ten days resulted in blood glucose levels twice as high as those in controls.[17] So be certain to tell your physician about both these studies and have him or her monitor you closely if you are interested in trying aloe along with your usual medications.

*Suggested Use:* If you have diabetes, do *not* try glyconutrients unless your doctor gives his or her okay. Not all diabetic patients respond to glyconutrient supplementation; in animals, aloe has been shown to raise as well as lower blood sugar. Diabetics interested in glyconutrient therapy need to work closely with their physicians to determine what dose of what glyconutrient is best. Start out slowly, with one glyconutrient at a time. Your doctor needs to monitor your insulin intake and blood sugar carefully to guard against hypoglycemia. Read labels carefully when purchasing glyconutrients. To enhance flavor, some manufacturers add extra sugar, which diabetics and those watching their weight should avoid.

## Juvenile Diabetes

Animal studies suggest that a strong initial response from an immune system well toned by glyconutrients may stave off the viruses thought to trigger the body's autoimmune reaction (coxsackie viruses in particular have been implicated) and prevent the onset of juvenile diabetes. In a recent study conducted at the University Hospital of Nijmegen in the Netherlands, for example, ling zhi-8, derived from reishi mushrooms, prevented the development of diabetes in mice with a predisposition to developing the disease.[18]

The cordyceps mushroom has also been tested in diabetic mice. In one controlled Japanese study at Gifu Pharmaceutical University, scientists injected male mice with a toxic chemical called streptozotocin, which destroyed their ability to produce insulin, thus bringing on a kind of type I diabetes. Controls received saline injections.[19] Then the mice received either cordyceps injections or the placebo injections. The cordyceps, unlike the placebo, resulted in a significant lowering of blood sugar, but not by stimulating insulin—these mice could no longer make the hormone. Instead, the cordyceps worked by increasing the activity of a liver enzyme responsible for the metabolism of glucose: glucokinase. The researchers also found that the cordyceps extracts normalized high blood sugar induced by epinephrine (adrenalin). In another study, some of the same researchers found that cordyceps extracts worked just as well in genetically diabetic mice.[20]

*Suggested Use:* As these are animal trials, scientists don't know if these glyconutrients will have the same effects on humans. Supplementing with glyconutrients, however, is a good way to strengthen your immune system. Diabetic patients interested in glyconutrient supplementation should take supplements only after consulting with their doctors to determine what amount and which glyconutrient is best. Your doctor needs to monitor your insulin intake and blood sugar carefully to guard against hypoglycemia. Read labels carefully when purchasing glyconutrients. To enhance flavor, some manufacturers add sweetener, which diabetics and those watching their weight should avoid. Start out slowly, with one glyconutrient at a time. Alternatively, you could add cooked mushrooms into your diet.

# Crohn's Disease, Interstitial Cystitis, Ulcerative Colitis, Irritable Bowel

Crohn's disease (chronic inflammation of the colon and ileum), ulcerative colitis (chronic inflammation and ulceration in the colon), and interstitial cystitis (chronic inflammation of the bladder) are considered autoimmune illnesses. Studies indicate that they may be caused by a defect in the body's mucosal-lining defensive barrier consisting of glycoproteins called glycosaminoglycans, or GAG for short.[21, 22] Wherever the barrier is defective— the bladder in interstitial cystitis, the colon in ulcerative colitis, and the ileum and colon in Crohn's—toxins and pathogens can penetrate, causing inflammation and infection. Fluid and protein leak out, disrupting the vascular structure and connective tissue. Chronic inflammation causes scarring and the body's shift into a high-gear immune response—and autoimmune disease.

What causes the GAG defect, which is often called leaky gut syndrome when the defect lies in the intestines, isn't clear. Genetics, toxins, diet, and pathogens may play a part. But rather than focusing on patching the leaky gut and restoring the body's balance, most treatments for Crohn's and ulcerative colitis concentrate on halting the body's inflammatory response, using steroids and other immune suppressants. Canadian researcher Alan L. Russell, however, believes that rebuilding the GAG layer may be more effective, theorizing that a degraded GAG layer sets the foundation for this cascade of infirmities.[23]

Lending support to his hypothesis is the fact that agents such as glucosamine and the synthetic polysaccharide Elmiron (used to treat interstitial cystitis) help reconstruct the GAG layer and often improve symptoms, whereas nonsteroidal anti-inflammatories like ibuprofen damage the GAG lining and exacerbate gut symptoms.[24] In addition, a diagnostic test for interstitial cystitis, which involves infusing potassium into the bladder, demonstrates that the potassium permeates the mucous barrier in many interstitial patients, causing pain. (In those without this condition, the potassium rarely causes pain.) Studies on rabbit bladders by researchers at the University of California at San Diego indicate that introducing polysaccharide compounds into the bladder decreases bladder permeability.[25]

Down the road, glucosamine may be a more practical GAG treatment for both bladder and gut. Researcher Russell suggests that low-dose heparin (a prescription blood thinner that's also a polysaccharide) as well as Elmiron may help rebuild the glycoprotein GAG barrier. Russell goes on to postulate that restoring the GAG layer may even help in rheumatoid arthritis. He notes that a drug called sulfasalazine, long used to treat ulcerative colitis, recently has been reclaimed for rheumatoid arthritis. It's believed to work by diminishing toxin absorption in the gut.[26]

Saccharide deficiencies have also been found in ulcerative colitis and Crohn's disease. As Dr. Neecie Moore details in her informative book *The Missing Link*, studies indicate that these patients are often deficient in fucose and N-acetylglucosamine; the latter simple sugar has also been used to treat damage that's already occurred.[27]

Other sugars may be affected in these illnesses as well. In 1981, researchers examined the mucus from the bowels of ten patients with Crohn's disease and compared it with that of normal controls.[28] More than half of the normal colons registered eight or more monosaccharides, whereas about a quarter of those with ulcerative colitis and Crohn's registered eight or more of these sugars.[29] What may help people with these disorders is *Aloe vera.* In a series of human trials, acemannan from aloe improved food digestion and absorption and enhanced "good" bacterial flora in the digestive tract, by reducing yeast and pH levels.[30]

Additionally, we know that gum sugars called arabinogalactans may help those with digestive tract problems, including irritable bowel. The glyconutrients are poorly digested and ferment in the large intestine. While this sounds like something better avoided, it's actually good: the fermentation produces short-chain fatty acids, crucial for preventing and alleviating diarrhea.[31] One of the most important of these fatty acids is called butyrate or butyric acid, a crucial metabolite for colon health.

*Suggested Use:* 500 milligrams to 1 gram of *Aloe vera* powdered extracts, in divided doses. Arabinogalactans: 250 milligrams to 1 gram daily, in divided doses. If you combine the glyconutrients, cut the amount for each in half. Any glyconutrient can cause gas, cramping, and diarrhea, particularly when you first begin, and people with inflammatory bowel disorders and irritable bowel may be more susceptible. If you experience any of these symptoms, cut back on the dose and take only with meals. Some evidence suggests that supplementing with 500 milligrams to 1 gram a day of vitamin C in divided doses along with the glyconutrients can relieve the symptoms.

Until human studies are conducted, it's too early to say if adding glucosamine will help symptoms of Crohn's disease, ulcerative colitis, or interstitial cystitis.

# Lupus

Lupus is an autoimmune connective-tissue disease that afflicts primarily women and is characterized by skin lesions, joint pain, arthritis, and kidney disease. Sometimes the nervous system is also affected and headaches, epilepsy, and psychosis can occur. Studies indicate that cordyceps mushrooms increase the survival of mice with lupus. In a controlled study by scientists in Taipei, Taiwan, mice fed a standardized extract from cordyceps daily for eight weeks had significant reduction in lymph-node size and an improvement in kidney function, and less protein in their urine, as compared with control animals.[32] Too much protein indicates kidney disease, which can progress to kidney failure—both of which can occur in lupus patients as well as in mice with the disease.

In addition, the cordyceps mice experienced a progressive reduction of what's called antinuclear antibodies (ANA for short), which are mounted in lupus against the body's own DNA. These antibodies are a hallmark of lupus: more than 98 percent of patients develop them. The Taipei scientists noted that while the effects of cordyceps in modulating the immune response were similar to those of cyclosporin—an immunosuppressive drug used to treat autoimmune diseases like lupus and to prevent organ-transplant rejection—the cordyceps, unlike the cyclosporin, was *not* toxic to the kidneys. In fact, the scientists continued, the mushroom was effective in *shielding* the kidney from the toxic effects of cyclosporin. For more information on treating the acute and chronic kidney problems that often accompany lupus and other diseases, read the Kidney Disease sections below. For more information on cordyceps's ability to inhibit cyclosporin-induced kidney damage in transplant patients, see the Transplant section.

# Kidney Disease

Many drugs, including antibiotics, chemotherapy, and antirejection drugs given to patients with lupus, arthritis, and transplanted organs, can rapidly injure the kidneys, resulting in *acute* kidney failure. *Chronic* renal (kidney) failure is the slow deterioration of kidney function and the end point of many diseases—from diabetes and lupus to certain viruses, heart disease, and drugs (both prescribed and recreational). In Western medicine, chronic renal failure is usually a one-way street toward dialysis, complete kidney failure, or kidney transplant. Western medications that treat chronic renal failure can only delay disease progression and address such accompanying problems as high blood pressure, bone loss, and anemia; they can't reverse the disease process.

Scientists at Shandong Medical University in China reported in a controlled study of fifty-one kidney-failure patients that the twenty-eight who received 3 to 5 grams of cordyceps extracts daily experienced improvements in both kidney and T-cell function, as compared with controls.[33] And in a 1998 review of a study of thirty-seven patients with renal disease, it was reported that 5 grams daily of the cordyceps extract Cs-4 for four weeks lowered kidney enzymes that spike in the illness and revved up the immune system by increasing superoxide dismutase (SOD), a blood enzyme that scavenges for free radicals.[34] Just as important, patients' symptoms subsided.

*Suggested Use:* If you have kidney disease, consult your doctor before trying glyconutrients. You will need to work closely with your physician to find the right amount of the right glyconutrient for you. Cordyceps has been proved effective, and anecdotally other glyconutrients have shown efficacy as well (see below). Cordyceps extracts or Cs-4: 3 to 6 grams in divided doses with water a half-hour before meals. Caution: Do not take cordyceps if you take a blood thinner or have a bleeding disorder unless under a doctor's care.

## KIDNEY DISEASE: A PATIENT'S SUCCESS

David is a forty-two-year-old business executive who's suffered from autoimmune chronic renal failure for several years. Though steroids controlled the inflammation in his kidneys for a while, his downward slide continued, and in 1995 he went on dialysis to help his body balance fluids and salts and excrete waste materials.

By the fall of 1997 David was getting dialysis three times a week because his kidney function was only 17 percent of normal. He needed a kidney transplant but no suitable donor was found, so he continued on dialysis. A few months later, on the suggestion of a friend, he started dietary supplementation with glyconutrients, a mixture of aloe extracts and arabinogalactans, 500 milligrams a day (see the resources chapter for more information). He continued to take this amount for about a year, and his kidney function stabilized.

Still tethered to his dialysis three times a week, David, with his doctor's approval, decided to increase the amount of glyconutrients to determine if higher doses would confer additional benefit. Over the course of a month he upped his intake to 12 to 18 grams a day. The first month, his kidney function increased from 17 percent to 32 percent. The second month it inched up to 37 percent, and by the end of the third month his kidney function had jumped to 68 percent, where it remained. His doctor no longer considers the kidney transplant necessary, but David still needs dialysis, twice a month. As you can see from David's story, glyconutrient intake is individual, and it often takes time to figure out what you need. It's important to work with a physician, particularly when contemplating the high intake of glyconutrients that David eventually settled into.

## Transplants

The immune-suppressant drug cyclosporin has been a boon to organ transplantation because it prevents organ rejection. It's problematic, however, because it's a potent renal toxin. Human and animal studies using the cordyceps mushroom show that the glyconutrient prevented, reduced, or reversed kidney damage by antibiotics and antirejection drugs.[35, 36] Equally crucial is that although cordyceps enhances immune functioning, it doesn't increase the rate of rejection of transplanted organs or tissue.

In a 1995 study of sixty-nine kidney-transplant patients, Chinese researchers found that kidney damage was significantly curtailed when cordyceps extract was added to the patients' cyclosporin therapy.[37] Controls who received cyclosporin alone sustained greater renal damage. Interestingly, the longer the administration time, the more significant the differences between the two groups, as far as kidney blood markers were concerned. The researchers recommended combining cyclosporin with cordyceps to mitigate kidney damage in kidney transplant recipients.

Even with immunosuppressant drugs, the body can reject transplanted tissue or organs as foreign—unless the donor is the identical twin of the recipient. Interestingly, animal studies and in vitro studies using human cells indicate that glyconutrients *decrease* the chances of tissue rejection—though we don't know how or why.[38] In rats, reishi extracts also delayed rejection of transplanted pancreatic islet cells, which are destroyed in diabetes. Down the road, such transplants may prove to be a viable treatment for the disease.

*Suggested Use:* If you have undergone a kidney transplant, consult your doctor before trying glyconutrients to diminish kidney damage conferred by antirejection drugs. With your doctor's okay, try 1 to 6 grams of cordyceps extract or Cs-4 daily, in divided doses. Start slowly and build up gradually.

The most striking feature about many chronic and autoimmune illnesses is that they can be managed with medications but rarely cured. People occasionally recover completely, but that's usually in spite of treatment. Most of the time the diagnosis is a life sentence of a waxing, waning disease. But glyconutrients have been shown to work without the deleterious side effects of drugs like steroids. Perhaps over the next hundred years the old adage for treatment with steroids will be changed to "When in doubt, use glyconutrients." That doesn't mean glyconutrients will supplant medications, but doctors and patients will be more conscious of using drugs as adjuncts to the body's own healing processes instead of as toxic treatments that destroy healthy tissues or that chronically paralyze the immune system. Glyconutrients, unlike many toxic drugs, empower the immune system, steadily steering it on a homeostatic course.

## Chapter 11

# Inhibiting Cancer

*Glyconutrients can improve both the odds of recovery and the quality of life in cancer patients. Glyconutrients also enhance standard chemotherapy and radiation and ease their debilitating side effects.*

In April, 1978, I was in my second year of medical school at Ibadan University, in Nigeria. Having completed a year and a half of intensive schooling in the basic sciences that underlie medicine, I had just started seeing my first real patients. Word came to us about a rare phenomenon occurring in the wards of our teaching hospital. The effects of the experience have remained with me ever since; indeed, I remember it as if it were yesterday.

An elderly woman had been admitted to our hospital with a diagnosis of thyroid cancer. But within a few days, and with no treatment, one of the residents noted that the patient's tumor had begun to shrink. Without chemotherapy, without radiation, without medical intervention of any kind, it continued to get smaller. Within a few weeks there was no trace of the malignancy that had brought her to the hospital.

What was most gratifying was that the patient experienced

no vomiting, no weight loss, no hair loss, no opportunistic infections—none of the unpleasant complications associated with the treatment of cancer. Although the woman was not my patient, I was among the steady stream of young medical students and doctors who shuffled up to the fourth floor to catch a glimpse of the miraculous lady. The mother of one of our internal medicine professors, she—and her son—were overjoyed at the outcome and as intrigued as everyone else by this unexpected event. Hers was a case of spontaneous remission of cancer, one of many medical terms for, "We don't know why this has happened, but we're glad that it did."

Fast-forward eight years to October 1986. It is 2 A.M., and I am with my own mother, who is dying of breast cancer. I try to ease her pain, placing my hands on her swollen belly and hugging her as best as I can. She had been treated two years before with surgery and radiation, but now the cancer has spread everywhere; her doctors have told me that there is nothing more they can do. Deep down, I know it is hopeless, but I keep trying to find hope. Tears pour down my face in the semidarkness of the hospital room. I feel helpless like a child by my mother's side. I don't know how to help her except in the most basic, human way—by showing her that I love her.

Doctors come face to face with death and often develop a defensive professional attitude to it. Other physicians had warned me that it feels different when your own family is affected. The most painful emotion for doctors is helplessness. That helplessness becomes a constant companion when we are unable to do anything of lasting value for many of the patients we encounter. When we help relieve someone's symptoms without addressing primary causes, the nagging feeling of having not done enough always remains. There is so much more of what we don't know than of what we do know.

As I stood by my mother's bedside I remembered the woman who experienced a spontaneous remission, and I wondered why it doesn't occur more often. Why wasn't my mother getting well? What prevents the immune system from waking up and taking care of business, as it ought to? Why do our bodies so often seem to function at a fraction of their intelligence? Do cultural blinders prevent us from seeing obvious and natural solutions? Is it just a matter of shifting focus?

My mother was not as lucky as the woman I encountered in medical school. She died on November 1, 1986. Since then, as I have gone about my business as a doctor and a student, I have kept one eye open for the secret of spontaneous remission. I know that its potential is within us and is innate to our bodies, but we remain blind to it somehow. Perhaps the elements of fear and desperation in our approach to treating cancer aggressively cause us to miss something obvious. The hope that we will discover what triggers these remissions has kept me in medicine.

The key to understanding spontaneous remission in cancer is appreciating that while it looks to be a highly unusual event, a miracle, it isn't: *it is the rule.* Every day normal people develop dozens of abnormal cells. Sunlight, viruses, bacteria, toxic chemicals, free radicals, poor nutrition, and genes all contribute to their development. Thousands of cells become malignant every year, but the body's vigilant immune system destroys them before they become full-blown cancers. When cancer develops, it means that some malignant cells have eluded detection and have established themselves. But even people with damaged immune systems generally do not end up with dozens of tumors of different kinds.

Cancerous, or neoplastic, cells have within them genes that fail to respond to normal restraints. The cells these genes inhabit divide on and on to form a tumor and eventually break free and spread, or metastasize. By the time we pinpoint the trouble with screening techniques, such as a mammogram in the case of breast cancer, the process has been ongoing for months or years and there are already billions of abnormal cells busily replicating.

The most efficient roles for glyconutrients in the diet are as broad-spectrum prevention, as nutritional protection, and as a means to increase the body's ability to sustain its structures and keep its identity intact. But when saccharides are added to the diet, it's been demonstrated that they can increase the efficiency of immune cells, whose job it is to scan the body for cancers and destroy them directly or call on other agents to assist.

If a cancer is already established, glyconutrients can, in some cases, arouse the immune system sufficiently to regress the tumor. You should always consult your doctor before trying glyconutrients if you have cancer: Some mushrooms and pectins have blood-thinning effects, and some cancer patients are vulnerable to bleeding problems, both from chemotherapy and from the cancer itself. However, my searches of the Chinese and Japanese literature did not reveal any studies or cases of abnormal bleeding resulting from the use of these mushrooms. You should *never* try to use glyconutrients as a sole treatment for your cancer—glyconutrients are nutritional supplements that work well with traditional therapies to help your body heal.

When embarking on glyconutrient supplementation for cancer, start slowly, and build up gradually over a few weeks. Take glyconutrients with a glass of water about a half hour before meals. If you experience cramping or diarrhea, cut back on the dose and build up more slowly; also consider taking the glyconutrients with meals. There is some evidence that supplementing with vitamin C (500 to 1,000 milligrams in divided doses) helps diminish gastrointestinal side effects. Those in remission should continue taking glyconutrients (see later in this chapter for information on which glyconutrients have been studied for particular cancers) to support the immune system, although the dose may be cut by 25 percent after the first year of remission. For patients being treated with radiation or chemotherapy, adding glyconutrients to the mix improves both the odds of recovery and the quality of life. See below for more on curbing the side effects of traditional cancer treatment, followed by information on specific cancers and the foods and extracts that have been used in clinical trials to treat them.

# Easing the Side Effects of Traditional Cancer Therapy

## CHEMOTHERAPY AND POLYSACCHARIDE K

Chemotherapy—the use of powerful drugs to kill cancer cells—is often highly toxic because it's not selective about which cells it kills. Many innocent, normal cells die along with the cancer cells. Glyconutrients enable the body to recover faster from the debilitating effects of chemo. Polysaccharide P, from the mushroom *Coriolus versicolor* and a close cousin of polysaccharide K, has been found to protect patients against the unpleasant side effects from chemotherapy and radiation as well as to relieve many of the same symptoms—pain, nausea, fatigue, cold sweats, and poor appetite—caused by the cancer itself. In doses up to 6 grams a day, the glyconutrient has proved successful in ameliorating side effects from several kinds of cancer in humans, including stomach, esophageal, and non-small-cell lung cancer.[1]

*Suggested Use:* After consulting with your doctor, try 1 to 6 grams of polysaccharide P daily, in divided doses. Start out at 500 milligrams and build up slowly. Children under twelve should not take polysaccharide P.

## CHEMOTHERAPY AND MAITAKE D-FRACTION

According to an expert at Kobe Pharmaceutical University in Japan, maitake extracts and maitake D-fraction not only inhibit cancer and its spread in cancer patients, but the glyconutrients also significantly reduce cancer pain and the side effects of chemotherapy.[2, 3, 4] In one trial of 165 participants with different, often advanced, cancers, 83 percent of those taking maitake reported a lessening of pain, and 90 percent reported a lessening of chemotherapy symptoms, including vomiting, nausea, reduced appetite, hair loss, intestinal bleeding, and lowered white count. Patients took 4 to 6 grams of maitake extract and 35 to 100 milligrams of maitake D-fraction in divided doses daily.

*Suggested Use:* Always consult with your doctor before beginning to take glyconutrients with your chemo. If you are allergic to mushrooms, do *not* try maitake mushrooms or extracts. Otherwise, 1 to 6 grams of maitake extract daily. For maitake D-fraction, 0.5 to 1.0 milligram per kilogram of body weight daily, in three divided doses. To find your weight in kilograms, multiply your weight in pounds by 0.45. For example, a 120-pound woman weighs 54 kilos and would take 27 to 54 milligrams of maitake D-fraction per day.

## CHEMOTHERAPY AND LENTINAN

5-Fluorouracil, better known as 5-FU, is a powerful drug used to treat many kinds of cancers, including breast, ovarian, and colon cancer, as well as other neoplasms of the digestive tract. One of its side effects is to shut down the bone marrow, preventing the production of the white cells, including neutrophils, macrophages, and lymphocytes—all critical to a healthy immune system. In mice, Japanese researchers found that intravenous lentinan (from the shiitake mushroom) prompted the rapid recovery of the white blood cells in the marrow and in the bloodstream.[5]

*Suggested Use:* As this is an animal study, we don't know if lentinan would bestow the same benefit on humans, but oral lentinan does enhance the workings of the immune system: 12.5 milligrams once or twice daily. Lentinan administered intramuscularly or intravenously is usually more effective than oral lentinan, but until human studies are done using the glyconutrient on these cancers, I cannot recommend injectable lentinan for this purpose. Injectable lentinan is available by prescription only and must be administered by a health-care professional. Serious side effects have occurred with IV lentinan, and they include fever, chills, back and leg pain, elevated liver enzymes, and anaphylaxis—a serious and potentially fatal allergic reaction.

## RADIATION AND GLYCONUTRIENTS

Active cells are killed easily by radiation, and as a general rule, cancer cells are active. But the process of killing cancer cells also damages or destroys normal tissue in the irradiated area. Radiation suppresses bone-marrow production and spleen function, leading to anemia and low white-cell counts—and thus to suppression of the immune system. Although the radiation itself is painless, the cancer patient may feel very sick in the days and weeks following the treatment as cells begin to swell and die and their contents break up into the body, which then endeavors to sweep up the damage.

Glyconutrients, including reishi and *Aloe vera,* have been found to decrease radiation sickness in animals and to help them recover faster.[6, 7, 8] Animals given these glyconutrients along with radiation gained weight faster and were less nauseated, and their blood counts returned to normal faster than did the counts of controls that were irradiated but did not receive glyconutrients. Topical preparations have also proved to be helpful. In one double-blind study on mice conducted at the renowned M.D. Anderson Cancer Center in Houston, Texas, a topical gel containing acemannan from aloe reduced skin reactions to radiation significantly.[9] The glyconutrient also increased the amount of radiation required to inflict skin damage. Researchers found that the gel was most effective if applied daily for at least two weeks immediately after each radiation treatment. The scientists found that the aloe didn't work if it was applied before irradiation or beginning one week after irradiation.

*Suggested Use:* It's too early to say if glyconutrients decrease radiation sickness in humans. The studies haven't been done, and therefore I cannot recommend that patients try glyconutrients until more is known.

## Alternatives to Supplements

Japanese researchers have found that whole edible mushrooms, including shiitake, maitake, and oyster—not just their extracts— are protective against bladder-induced cancers in mice caused by a chemical toxin.[10] The scientists treated sixty-seven mice with a carcinogen called BBN every day for eight weeks. Ten of the mice received only BBN. The rest received BBN and mushrooms. All ten mice treated with BBN alone developed bladder cancer. But the mice that ate mushrooms along with the BBN fared significantly better: About half of them developed cancer. In addition, in the ten mice treated with BBN alone, both macrophage and natural killer activity were significantly depressed, whereas those immune system markers registered nearly normal in the mushroom-treated groups. As with the extracts, the whole mushroom worked by boosting the activity of the immune system's white blood cells rather than by directly killing cells.

*Suggested Use:* No human studies have been done using whole mushrooms to treat bladder cancer, but adding shiitake, maitake, and oyster mushrooms is a good way to bring glyconutrients to your diet. As long as you know you are not allergic to mushrooms, I'd recommend cooked shiitake, maitake, and oyster mushrooms twice a day—about a handful of mushrooms at each serving. For a recipe for preparing mushroom tea, see the resources chapter.

## Cancers

### BLADDER CANCER

In a small human study, oral administration of 3 grams of polysaccharide K to patients with bladder cancer daily for seven days prior to surgery resulted in an increased ability of killer white cells to eradicate cancer cells in five of the ten patients studied.[11] In addition, some animal studies indicate that polysaccharide K enhances the effectiveness of the chemotherapy agent carboquone, resulting in less weight loss and increased inhibition of both tumor growth and spread to the lungs (where bladder cancer often metastasizes).[12]

*Suggested Use:* Try 3 grams daily of polysaccharide K, in divided doses. Start out at 500 milligrams with this glyconutrient, and build up slowly. Occasionally polysaccharide K causes a benign darkening of the fingernails.

## BREAST CANCER

Studies in humans with breast cancer suggest that polysaccharide K may convey additional benefit to standard chemotherapy, radiation therapy, and endocrine therapy with tamoxifen, an estrogen blocker, used to treat the disease.

Polysaccharide K seems particularly helpful when a tumor protein marker called HLA B40 registers positive in the breast tumor. (HLA stands for histocompatibility locus antigen.) When breast tumors register a particular HLA antigen called B40, it usually signifies a more favorable prognosis. Researchers at Gunma University School of Medicine in Japan found that when B40-positive patients took standard chemotherapy plus 3 grams of polysaccharide K a day for two months a year for five years, the 10-year survival rate was 100 percent.[13] That's in contrast to the controls, the B40-positive patients who received only standard chemotherapy: Their survival rate was 84 percent.

While the B40-negative patients didn't fare nearly as well as either of the B40-positive groups, those on polysaccharide K did do better over ten years. However, at five years, those on chemotherapy alone did marginally better: the survival rate was 82 percent on chemo alone versus 76 percent for those on chemo plus polysaccharide K.

Part of the problem with using saccharides to treat breast cancer, or indeed any cancer, is that saccharides aren't tried until other measures have failed—they tend to be used in desperate, last-ditch efforts, and by that time the cancer is advanced and more resistant to treatment. Earlier intervention in cancers, as with most other serious illnesses, generally yields more favorable results. Breast-cancer studies with C3H/OuJ mice, a breed that develops breast tumors spontaneously, support this fact. In a Japanese study, these tumor-prone mice were divided into two groups of forty. Both groups received a normal diet, but one group had polysaccharide K added to its feed. Within fifteen weeks, both tumor incidence and number were significantly lower in the polysaccharide group, as compared with controls, and survival rates also improved.[14]

Along similar lines, in another Japanese study, researchers fed female rats a cancer-causing agent called DMBA. Some also received polysaccharide K daily in addition to the cancer-causing agent. It took significantly longer for the polysaccharide K-fed rats to develop breast tumors than for the control rats.[15] Just as important, response to treatment with tamoxifen significantly improved in those rats that received polysaccharide K.

Maitake D-fraction has also proved significantly helpful in animal studies on breast cancer. In one study, researchers at Japan's Kobe Pharmaceutical University implanted breast cancer cells in young mice; the tumors were later removed.[16] Then the investigators injected half the mice with maitake D-fraction daily for ten days, while the controls received a placebo injection of saline. After twenty days, 100 percent of the control group had developed breast tumors and metastasis, whereas only 8 percent of the maitake mice had breast tumors and 7 percent had metastasis.

*Suggested Use:* Always consult your doctor before starting on glyconutrients: 3 to 6 grams of polysaccharide K, in divided doses. Start out at 500 milligrams with this glyconutrient, and build up slowly. Maitake D-fraction: see Chemotherapy and Maitake D-fraction section earlier in the chapter for intake information based on human results. If you combine two glyconutrients, cut your dose for each in half.

## COLON CANCER: A PATIENT'S SUCCESS

I first met seventy-five-year-old Fredericka at her rural farmhouse in the spring of 1997. A few months earlier, she had had surgery for colon cancer. Unfortunately, Fredericka's cancer was caught very late, and surgeons were able to remove only some of the tumor and perform a colostomy. The cancer had also spread to the liver, where colon cancer usually travels first. Fredericka had been employed as a school administrator for many years but was too ill to continue working at the school she loved. But the day I met her, she was sitting up and receiving phone calls from students and teachers, still helping them resolve problems. They welcomed her sensible advice and her kind, reassuring voice. Fredericka had a strong will and a sharp wit.

But her body was failing her. Fredericka was already rail thin, and her cheeks were sunken. A hospice patient, she had the wasted look common in people with advanced cancer. Fredericka had opted against chemotherapy or radiation. She had had a full life, she told me, and didn't want to suffer more from the treatment than from the disease itself. She did agree to pain medication and gentler alternative measures, including nutritional supplementation, massage therapy, and a therapeutic-touch method of healing called Reiki. Without chemotherapy and radiation, her life expectancy was about two months.

I suggested to Fredericka that she add a mixture of arabino-galactans and a stabilized aloe extract in powder form to her regimen. (See the resources section for more information.) Over a week or so, she gradually upped her dosage to 3 grams daily in divided doses. About a month after starting on the protocol, her appetite began to perk up and she gained weight. In all, she gained about 30 pounds. Her sunken cheeks filled out, and her energy improved. She was able to take care of her own grooming needs and cook an occasional meal—a significant improvement in her quality of life. Fredericka continued doing well for eighteen months; she died in her sleep in her own bed at the age of 77. Did glyconutrients account for her improved, longer-than-expected life span? Studies suggest that the saccharides may indeed have contributed.

## COLORECTAL AND STOMACH CANCERS

Promising Japanese studies on colorectal cancer suggest that polysaccharide K may improve the chances of survival. In a study at the Kyushu University School of Medicine, after two groups of patients totaling 111 had surgery for colorectal cancer, one group of 56 patients received polysaccharide K (3 grams a day for two months, then 2 grams a day for two years, then 1 gram a day thereafter), and the other group of 55 patients received a placebo.[17] The study was double blind—meaning that neither the scientists nor the patients knew who was getting the glyconu-trient and who was getting the dummy drug. Patients had advanced disease, stages III and IV. (In contrast, in stages I and II, the cancers are caught earlier and are less invasive.) Both groups were followed for eight years. Of the polysaccharide K patients, 40 percent survived, versus 25 percent of controls. The glyconutrients also affected the disease-free period of time: 25 percent of the polysaccharide K patients were disease-free at eight years, compared with only 8 percent of controls.[18, 19]

*Suggested Use:* Always consult your doctor before starting on glyconutrients. Polysaccharide K: 1 to 6 grams a day in divided doses. Start out at 500 milligrams with this glyconutrient and build up slowly. Arabinogalactans: 2 to 3 grams a day. *Aloe vera* powdered extract: 500 to 1,000 milligrams a day, in divided doses. Or liquid *Aloe vera*: 2 to 4 ounces a day, in divided doses. The liquid form of *Aloe vera* is more likely to cause cramping and diarrhea. Cut back or discontinue should either occur. If you are combining two glyconutrients, cut the dose for each by half; if you combine three glyconutrients, cut the dose for each by two-thirds.

In a controlled studies on humans, adding 1 milligram of intravenous lentinan twice weekly or 2 milligrams of IV lentinan once weekly to traditional treatment protocols showed impressive results in increasing survival rates and improving the quality of life of people with advanced and recurrent stomach cancer and colorectal cancer.[20, 21, 22] Researchers found that T cells and macrophages mediated the glyconutrients' antitumor effects. Obviously, using IV lentinan must be done with your physician's approval and administered by a qualified health professional.

Lentinan is better absorbed and more effective intravenously than orally. Serious side effects have occurred with IV lentinan, and they include fever, chills, back and leg pain, elevated liver enzymes, and anaphylaxis—a serious and potentially fatal allergic reaction. Doses are calculated by your doctor according to your weight and health status. (See the resources section for more information.)

## ESOPHAGEAL CANCER

Researchers at the Cooperative Study Group for Esophageal Cancer in Japan followed 158 esophageal cancer patients for five years.[23] Patients were placed in one of four groups. One group received chemotherapy, the second group received chemotherapy and 3 grams daily of polysaccharide K, the third group received only polysaccharide K, and the fourth group served as the controls. Patients on polysaccharide K and chemotherapy had a significantly better survival rate at five years than did those on chemotherapy alone.

*Suggested Use:* Always get your doctor's approval before adding glyconutrients to your medical treatment. Try 3 to 6 grams of polysaccharide K daily, in divided doses. Start out at 500 milligrams with this glyconutrient, and build up slowly.

## LEUKEMIA

In a 1981 study at the School of Medicine at Tokai University near Tokyo, researchers administered polysaccharide K along with standard chemotherapy to fourteen patients with acute leukemia; 14 other patients served as the controls and received only standard chemotherapy.[24] The scientists found that complete remissions were longer in the polysaccharide K patients. In addition, the average survival time for those on polysaccharide K was twenty-one months, as compared with twelve months for the controls. Only one of the controls is still alive, as compared with three polysaccharide patients. Of course, standard chemotherapy for leukemia has come a long way since this 1981 study. It would be interesting to see survival statistics from a study conducted today with the more advanced chemotherapies plus polysaccharide K.

*Suggested Use:* Always consult with your doctor before adding glyconutrients to your medical treatment. Try 3 grams of polysaccharide K, in divided doses. Start out at 500 milligrams with this glyconutrient, and build up slowly.

## LIVER CANCER

Liver or hepatic cancer is one of the fastest progressing and most virulent cancers. Active hexose correlated compound (AHCC), derived from the shiitake mushroom, increases survival times and quality of life for people with liver cancer caused by hepatitis C, a common cause of hepatic cancer.[25] In a 1999 Japanese study of 126 patients, forty-four received 3 grams of AHCC daily, while eighty-two received a placebo after surgery. After one year the AHCC patients registered a significantly higher survival rate than the control group. In addition, key blood markers indicated that liver damage dropped, while white-cell and red-cell counts rose. Patients also reported an increase in appetite. However, whereas survival, blood work, and quality of life improved in the AHCC group, tumor recurrence did *not* decline. Curiously, although the AHCC patients with hepatitis C did survive longer, those who didn't have hepatitis or those with hepatitis B (another cause of liver cancer) did not experience better survival rates.

Other liver cancer studies involving people have been less optimistic. In a study at Hirosaki University School of Medicine in Japan, researchers found that polysaccharide K and lentinan in combination with the standard chemotherapy drug 5-FU provided no additional benefit in prolonging life or the quality of life over the 5-FU alone.[26]

A professor at Kobe Pharmaceutical University has focused a great deal of animal research on maitake D-fraction's ability to prevent liver cancer. In one study, he injected liver cancer cells into mice. One group of mice then received maitake powder in their feed, another group received maitake injections, and the third group served as controls. After thirty days, the scientist found that 100 percent of the controls had developed liver cancer, as compared with 19 percent of the maitake-fed mice and 9 percent of the maitake-injected mice.[27]

Next the professor added the chemical N-nitrosodi-n-butylamine, which induces liver cancer, to the diet of three groups of mice. Again, one group received maitake powder orally, another group received maitake injections, and the third group served as controls. Results were similar to those in the first trial: One hundred percent of the controls developed liver cancer, versus 22 percent of the maitake-fed mice and less than 10 percent of the maitake-injected mice.[28]

In another study, the professor investigated the effects of maitake D-fraction injections in combination with the traditional chemotherapy drug Mitomycin C.[29] After injecting liver cancer into mice, he divided the mice into two groups: the Mitomycin-only mice versus the Mitomycin-with-maitake-D-fraction mice. Following ten days of therapy, he found that the D-fraction potentiated the Mitomycin significantly. About half of the Mitomycin-only mice developed metastasis, versus only 13 percent of the mice that received both Mitomycin and maitake D-fraction.

The key to efficacy may be in the timing. As stated earlier, glyconutrients tend to work better in preventing problems than in treating them. When, for instance, scientists administered polysaccharide K to hamsters before injecting these lab animals with a liver cancer-causing agent called Thorotrast, the cancer incidence was reduced by about half—and the lives of the hamsters that developed cancer were prolonged.[30]

*Suggested Use:* Always consult with your doctor before adding glyconutrients to your medical treatment. Try 3 to 6 grams of AHCC daily, in divided doses.

## LUNG CANCER

Lung cancer is one of the deadliest cancers, and it's often not caught until late in the disease process. Five-year survival studies were conducted at Gunma University School of Medicine in Japan on lung-cancer patients after radiation therapy resulted in complete or partial shrinkage of the tumor. Of the 225 patients in the study, 170 had squamous cell lung cancer. Half of the group was randomly assigned to receive 3 grams of polysaccharide K in cycles of two weeks on and two weeks off, while the other half, the control group, received a dummy drug. Survival in the polysaccharide K group was significantly longer than in the control group.[31] Patients in the study were classified as stage I-II or stage III. (Again, in stage III, the disease is more advanced than in stage I or II.) The five-year survival rates of patients on glyconutrients with stages I-II and stage III disease were 39 percent and 26 percent, respectively, while the controls' rates were 17 percent and 8 percent. In the world of oncology, that's a big difference.

*Suggested Use:* Always consult your doctor before starting on glyconutrients. Administering polysaccharide K in cycles of two weeks on and two weeks off has not been proved to be more effective than daily dosing with 3 grams in divided doses. Start out at 500 milligrams with this glyconutrient, and build up slowly.

## LYMPHOMA

Lymphomas are solid tumors of white blood cells called lymphocytes; Jacqueline Kennedy Onassis and King Hussein of Jordan both died from a form of the disease called non-Hodgkins's lymphoma. Viruses have been implicated in causing lymphoma in humans, and we know viruses can cause the disease in animals. Laboratory mice infected with certain viruses, for instance, develop lymphomas quickly. Colleagues at Hebrew University-Hadassah Medical School in Jerusalem showed that polysaccharide K delayed the onset of lymphoma in mice inoculated with a lymphoma-causing virus.[32, 33] Although it couldn't protect the mice from the disease, polysaccharide K did slow down the progression of the lymphoma and caused infected cells to die. In addition, the glyconutrients also increased activity of cytotoxic T cells, which in turn destroyed the abnormal cells.

*Suggested Use:* Although human trials have yet to be conducted on polysaccharide K and lymphoma, the glyconutrient has been found safe and effective in other human cancers and may be worth trying together with traditional medical treatment. Consult your doctor before trying polysaccharide K. Children under 12 should not take the glyconutrient. Follow the manufacturer's suggestions and your doctor's advice.

## NASOPHARYNGEAL CANCER

Nasopharyngeal cancer is cancer of the pharynx, which is located directly behind the nasal passages. In a 1989 study conducted at Machay Memorial Hospital in Taipei, thirty-eight patients with nasopharyngeal cancer received radiation and a course of standard chemotherapy. Next, investigators gave patients either 3 grams of polysaccharide K or a placebo daily. Survival for the polysaccharide patients was 28 percent after five years, as compared with 15 percent for controls.[34] These findings echo those of an earlier study by some of the same scientists.[35]

*Suggested Use:* Always consult your doctor before starting on glyconutrients. Try 3 grams of polysaccharide K daily, in divided doses. Start out at 500 milligrams with this glyconutrient and build up slowly.

### PROSTATE CANCER

Prostate cancer used to be a subject men shied away from discussing, but as prominent men—actor Sidney Poitier, Senator Bob Dole, retired general Norman Schwarzkopf, junk-bond king Michael Milken, New York Mayor Rudy Giuliani, and comedian Jerry Lewis, among them—have begun opening up about their own experiences with the disease, the stigma has slowly lifted. Prostate cancer is the second most common cause of cancer death in men, after lung cancer, and is more prevalent in blacks than whites. Prostate cancer can be slowly progressive or virulent; the latter scenario occurs more often in younger men, with the disease claiming the life of musician Frank Zappa at age fifty-three and actor Bill Bixby at fifty-nine.

I've heard two compelling anecdotes of patients with prostate cancer who've benefited from glyconutrients. In April 1996, Frank, a sixty-five-year-old art professor, began experiencing difficulty urinating. Frank's family physician referred him to a urologist, who found a large tumor on physical examination. A blood test called a prostate specific antigen (PSA) test confirmed the diagnosis of prostate cancer. Frank had a particularly aggressive form of the disease, and his tumor was too large to remove. Instead, he was immediately started on radiation and chemotherapy, but the tumor continued to grow. Seven months later, he decided to start supplementing with rice bran, rich in beta-glucans and the polysaccharide arabinoxylane, which has been shown to promote natural killer cell activity in test-tube studies.[36] Frank took 1 gram three times a day, and within four months the tumor had shrunk sufficiently to be removed surgically. A year after surgery, he halved his rice-bran intake and has remained on it and in remission for four years.

When forty-nine-year-old Emmanuel went for his annual physical exam, his doctor felt a small nodule on his prostate gland. His initial PSA reading was very high at 112 (0–5 is normal). Distraught because he had a young family and a peaking career and couldn't face dealing with the possible consequences of his illness, including impotence and urinary incontinence, Emmanuel decided against traditional medical treatment and instead, after conferring with a friend, tried glyconutrients. He took 3 grams of powdered aloe extracts daily. Four weeks later his PSA was 11; six weeks later it had dropped to 3, and, on examination, the nodule had disappeared.

While Emmanuel's story had a happy ending, not everyone responds to glyconutrients, and in any event, we can't be sure that Emmanuel did respond—his could have been the rare case of spontaneous remission. Furthermore, glyconutrients often work synergistically with traditional therapy; it should not be a matter of choosing one over the other. Human studies using *Aloe vera* or rice bran to treat prostate cancer have not been done, so I can't recommend either Emmanuel's or Frank's protocols until more is known.

To help improve immune functioning, however, supplementing with aloe extracts or rice bran is a good idea. Read rice-bran labels carefully; doses vary. To enhance flavor, some manufacturers add sweetener, which diabetics and those watching their weight should avoid.

Animal studies do indicate that glyconutrients are effective in treating prostate cancer. National Institute of Health Swiss athymic mice (they have no thymus gland) are a breed of laboratory animal that lack T cells—white blood cells vital to immune system functioning. At the University of North Carolina at Chapel Hill, researchers found that polysaccharide K reduced the rate of growth of human prostate cancer cells injected into these mice, particularly when the cancer was caught early.[37] Polysaccharide K also increased host survival and decreased the incidence and number of cancerous lesions in the lung, to which prostate cancer often spreads.

These researchers also tried polysaccharide K on athymic Beige mice. Unlike the Swiss mice, Beige mice are deficient in natural killer cells as well as T cells, and unfortunately, the Beige mice did not reap the same benefits in the study. Despite glyconutrient supplementation, the cancers spread rapidly. This finding suggests that natural killer cell activity is critical in fighting tumor growth and metastasis—and glyconutrients also boost activity of these cells.[38, 39, 40, 41] In another prostate cancer study at the University of North Carolina, this time on rats, researchers found that although polysaccharide K didn't reverse prostate cancer on its own, it did enhance the effects of standard chemotherapy by improving survival, retarding growth locally, decreasing metastasis, and prolonging life.[42] Moreover, the researchers postulated that polysaccharide K may enhance the effects of standard chemotherapeutic agents in resistant prostate cancer.

Like polysaccharide K, pectins reduce prostate-cancer metastasis in animals. In one study, rats with prostate cancer that received pectin had significantly fewer lung metastases than did control rats.[43] In addition, urologists at New York Medical College recently reported that a beta-glucan extract of maitake mushrooms killed prostatic cancer cells in the test tube, an effect potentiated by vitamin C and the cancer drug carmustine.[44]

*Suggested Use:* Until human studies are conducted, we won't know if pectins and polysaccharide K are effective in treating prostate cancer. Taking one or both of the glyconutrients to boost overall immunity, however, may be helpful. Consult with your doctor before trying either glyconutrient. Follow manufacturer's recommendations or your doctor's advice.

## SARCOMA

Several glyconutrients have been tested on sarcomas—malignancies that spring from cells of connective tissue, including muscle, cartilage, and bone. In fact, there are more than fifty articles on the medical computer database Medline that address the use of saccharides to treat sarcomas—many with promising results. Following in the footsteps of Dr. William Coley a hundred years before, Texas researchers in 1991 injected acemannan from aloe straight into the tumors of 43 cats and dogs.[45] Of those animals, twenty-six showed evidence of their immune system attacking the tumors, and twelve showed significant clinical improvement, assessed by tumor shrinkage, tumor necrosis (meaning the tumor shriveled up and was destroyed), and prolonged survival. Five of the seven animals with fibrosarcomas, which arise from the fibrous connective tissue, were among the twelve that improved.

Japanese researchers at Tokyo's National Cancer Center Hospital demonstrated that extracts of sarcodon and reishi mushrooms are also effective against sarcomas in animals.[46] Other researchers suggest that polysaccharide extracts of reishi and murill mushrooms as well as *Aloe vera* are effective against sarcomas.[47, 48, 49] When scientists tested an aloe polysaccharide on melanoma and sarcoma tumors in mice, they found that it effected cures only in fibrosarcoma tumors. However, the growth rate of other tumors slowed down in the treated mice, unlike in the controls.[50]

*Suggested Use:* Because these are animal studies, we don't know if *Aloe vera* or sarcodon, reishi, or murill mushrooms are effective in treating sarcoma in people, but aloe and mushrooms are potent immune boosters. Before adding glyconutrients to boost immunity, always consult your doctor. To enhance overall immunity, try 500 to 1,000 milligrams a day of *Aloe vera* powdered extract, in divided doses. Or liquid *Aloe vera*: 2 to 4 ounces a day, in divided doses. Caution: The liquid form of *Aloe vera* is more likely to cause cramping and diarrhea. Cut back or discontinue should either occur. Sarcodon, reishi, or murill extracts: 3 to 6 grams a day, in divided doses.

If you combine two glyconutrients, cut the dose for each by half; if you add three, cut the dose for each by two-thirds. Caution: Reishi mushrooms contain a substance that thins the blood and can cause bleeding. Do not take reishi mushrooms if you take a blood thinner or have a bleeding disorder without consulting a physician.

## SKIN CANCER

Gus is a fifty-year-old lab technician who presented in 1999 with a bleeding malignant melanoma, the most serious form of skin cancer, on his back. Tests revealed that the cancer had already metastasized to distant lymph nodes, skin, and bone, and that the tumor was particularly aggressive. After the local tumor was surgically removed, Gus was started on chemotherapy and placed on interferon to help jump-start his immune system. The interferon made him very sick and he asked to be taken off the drug. Besides, it wasn't working: The melanoma continued to grow. (Many melanoma patients do not respond favorably to traditional chemotherapy.) On his doctor's advice Gus decided to try glyconutrients, including aloe extracts (12 grams daily) and yeast beta-glucans (100 milligrams daily). After one month the metastases began to shrink on CAT scan. A year later Gus was in remission and taking 4 grams of aloe extracts daily, plus the yeast beta-glucans. He went back to work feeling healthy and well.

Recent animal studies suggest that glyconutrients may improve survival and inhibit the metastasis of melanoma in mice by increasing T-cell and macrophage activity against the melanoma cells.[51, 52] In one study, researchers at Tokyo Women's Medical College discovered that by increasing neutrophil action, polysaccharide K decreased the size and the number of liver-cancer cells that spread to the lungs in mice.[53] In another study, polysaccharide K suppressed, both in vitro (in the test tube) and in vivo (in the organism), melanoma metastasis in mice.[54] Cordyceps is also effective. In one study, IV injections of cordyceps extract into mice with melanoma resulted in an increase of natural killer cells, key players in the immune response, and a decrease in metastasis to the lungs.[55]

*Suggested Use:* Human studies using glyconutrients to treat melanoma haven't been conducted; until we know more, I can't recommend Gus's protocol. However, adding *Aloe vera* extracts and yeast beta-glucans to your diet to increase your immunity is a good idea. Follow the manufacturer's recommended doses or your doctor's advice.

We don't know if polysaccharide K can treat skin cancer in humans, but in other cancers the glyconutrient has been shown to be effective: 3 grams of polysaccharide K, in divided doses. Start out at 500 milligrams with this glyconutrient, and build up slowly. To boost general immunity, cordyceps extracts: 3 to 6 grams a day, in divided doses. Caution: Cordyceps contains a substance that thins the blood and can potentially cause bleeding. Patients who take blood thinners or have a bleeding disorder should not take cordyceps without their doctor's okay.

### STOMACH CANCER

Stomach cancer is far more common in Japan than in the United States, and Japanese scientists are focused on uncovering the causes of this disease. Published in the journal *Lancet,* a 1994 Japanese study of 262 patients with stomach cancer concluded that the five-year survival rate of the group given 3 grams of polysaccharide K plus chemotherapy was significantly higher than the rate for those on chemotherapy alone.[56] The five-year disease-free rate was also substantially greater in the polysaccharide K-treated group. In general, the more advanced the gastric cancer, the lower the patient's immunity. Other studies indicate that cell-mediated immunity is restored if the patient receives polysaccharide K or lentinan.[57, 58]

In another study, researchers treated stage III stomach cancer patients with polysaccharide K or placebo after surgery.[59] Although polysaccharide K extended the disease-free period over eighty months, survival was not significantly extended. The self-critical researchers chastised themselves for their tentative dosing of 3 grams daily for the first two months, then 2 grams daily for up to fourteen months, followed by 1 gram daily for the remainder of the trial. Had the dosage remained at 3 grams daily, the scientists theorized, results would have been more encouraging. No significant side effects were observed, except for a darkening of the fingernails in four of the seventy-seven patients.

*Suggested Use:* Always consult your doctor before starting on glyconutrients. Try 3 grams of polysaccharide K, in divided doses. Start out at 500 milligrams with this glyconutrient, and build up slowly.

# In Brief: Other Human Cancer Studies Using Glyconutrients

## POLYSACCHARIDE K

In a review article, a 1992 double-blind Chinese trial is described in which 274 patients with stomach, esophageal, or lung cancer received chemotherapy and radiation plus either 3 grams of polysaccharide P or shark liver oil daily (another immune booster, shark liver oil is rich in omega-3 fatty acids, the active component in fish oils).[60] Effectiveness was calculated on improvement in blood profiles, including white count, and significant increase in weight or the ability to care for oneself. At the end of the six-month trial the scientists broke the code and found that polysaccharide P was effective 82 percent of the time, versus 45 percent for the shark liver oil.

*Suggested Use:* Always consult your doctor before adding glyconutrients to your treatment protocol. Try 3 grams of polysaccharide P, in divided doses. Start out at 500 milligrams with this glyconutrient, and build up slowly.

## BOVINE TRACHEAL CARTILAGE

Rich in saccharides, bovine tracheal cartilage has shown efficacy in several types of hard-to-treat cancers, including those of the brain, pancreas, lung, and ovary. Animal and human studies at Hershey Medical Center and elsewhere suggest that the glyconutrient may improve the immune response against many kinds of solid tumors, particularly kidney cancer, which is usually resistant to conventional treatment once it has spread.[61, 62] In particular, the glyconutrient has been shown to shrink metastases in the lung, to which kidney cancer often spreads.

*Suggested Use:* Always consult your doctor before starting on glyconutrients. Try 6 to 9 grams daily of bovine tracheal cartilage, in divided doses. Start at 1 gram, and build up gradually. The risk of contracting mad cow disease from bovine tracheal cartilage, while unlikely, has not been scientifically disproved. For more information, see chapter 2.

## ALOE VERA

In a 1998 study conducted in Milan, Italy, twenty-six patients with advanced solid tumors (including cancers of the breast, gastrointestinal tract, brain, and lung) who hadn't responded to traditional therapy were treated daily with 20 milligrams of melatonin, which has been shown to induce some benefits in untreatable metastatic cancer patients. Another twenty-four patients received 20 milligrams of melatonin daily plus a tincture (alcohol-based liquid) of *Aloe vera*, 1 milliliter twice a day.[63] A partial response was achieved in two of the twenty-four patients treated with melatonin plus aloe, whereas none of the patients treated with melatonin alone improved. In addition, the cancer stabilized in fourteen of the aloe patients, compared with only seven of the melatonin patients.

*Suggested Use:* Always consult your doctor before starting on glyconutrients. There is no advantage to a using a tincture over powdered or liquid *Aloe vera*, and many people can't tolerate the alcohol. Aloe powdered extract: 500 to 1,000 milligrams a day, in divided doses. Liquid *Aloe vera*: 2 to 4 ounces a day, in divided doses. Caution: The liquid form of *Aloe vera* is more likely to cause cramping and diarrhea. Cut back or discontinue should either occur. If you are combining two glyconutrients, cut the dose for each by half.

Although hundreds of studies have pointed to the efficacy of glyconutrients in treating many kinds of cancers, it's important to note that glyconutrients are just one part of effective treatment. Whatever treatment a cancer patient undergoes, good nutrition is essential. Of course, it's tough to eat right when radiation and chemotherapy are making you sick. Again, that's where glyconutrients are beneficial, easing many of those miserable side effects.

## Chapter 12

# Fighting Hepatitis, HIV, and Opportunistic Infections

*How glyconutrients help treat serious viral and bacterial infections.*

**C**indy, a family therapist and teacher living in Indianapolis, was infected with the hepatitis C virus when she was two days old—what she calls an "unwanted gift" from a well-intentioned stranger who donated the blood used to treat her severe jaundice. Though she began experiencing symptoms in her early twenties, she wasn't diagnosed until 1997, when she was thirty-three. The side effects she's endured from treatment with interferon A—a cytokine that fights viruses and is often used to treat hepatitis B and C—have been severe, and she detailed them in an up-front article for the magazine *Indianapolis Monthly*.[1] Her symptoms, she writes, began several hours after her first dose: "At 3 A.M., all hell broke loose. I made a beeline for the bathroom and, in the nick of time, lost the day's meals in the sink. . . . I headed to the computer for some newsgroup comfort. The message came back loud and clear: Welcome to our world.

"The side effects compounded over the next few days: fatigue and insomnia (an ironically nasty combo), nausea, chills, head-aches, and intense irritability. I remember telling my husband—outside of the earshot of my kids—that there was no way I could do this. As much as I tried, I couldn't hide the effects from my family. . . . They asked about the biohazard needle discard container in my bathroom. They helped make room for my $1,600-a-month interferon stash around the juices and cheese sticks in the refrigerator. For a school project, my daughter Emily was asked what three wishes she would have for her family. She wrote: 'I only have one wish. That is for my mom to get better.' "

Glyconutrients offer new hope to hepatitis sufferers because these nutrients have been shown to optimize the production of interferons locally—exactly where they are needed—so there's none of the toxicity Cindy encountered. When interferons are produced naturally in a healthy person, they are released in much smaller quantities, so reactions like Cindy's don't usually occur. That doesn't mean nature's interferons aren't powerful or effective. Quite the contrary: they're more effective because they're released exactly where and when they are needed. They improve natural killer cell function, antibody production, T-cell activity, and macrophage efficiency without inducing massive, nonspecific immune stimulation, as the interferons given to patients like Cindy do.

In this way, glyconutrients offer an advantage over drugs, which often rev up the immune system without inciting a massive immune response that usually makes its recipients feel very sick, as if they have a terrible case of the flu. Interestingly, people taking glyconutrients show no evidence of increased activity of their immune cells in between challenges to the immune system. When confronted with viruses or bacteria, however, the immune system gears up quickly and highly specifically to the particular challenge. That doesn't mean we should substitute glyconutrients for interferon and other standard drugs. It does mean that in many cases glyconutrients are useful adjuncts to current treatment protocols.

## Hepatitis B and C

Hepatitis B and C are serious public health problems around the world. Although the public knows more about hepatitis B, thanks in part to the candor of celebrities Naomi Judd, Kenny Rogers, and Evel Knievel, who've contracted it, hepatitis C, in fact, affects more people and is much more likely to become chronic. The Centers for Disease Control in Atlanta estimates that more than a million Americans are infected with hepatitis B (communicated by sexual contact or blood) and 3.9 million have hepatitis C (primarily blood-borne). About 75 percent of those infected with hepatitis C will develop chronic infections.

In hepatitis B, the numbers are lower—only 6 to 10 percent. (Hepatitis A, spread by fecal-oral contact, rarely becomes chronic.) We don't know exactly why some people recover and others don't, and chronic hepatitis can smolder for years. But we do know that those with persistent problems have a faulty immune response to the virus. Instead of effectively eliminating the pathogen, their bodies go into a kind of stalemate between the virus and the immune system, with the liver as the battleground. The inflamed, battle-weary liver becomes scarred, and immune functioning is poor.

Hepatitis B and C are sometimes called stealth viruses; they're relatively quiet viruses that often dodge notice by the immune system. Surreptitiously they attach their own DNA to that of the victim and busily replicate undisturbed in the host's DNA as the cells divide. In time, multiple copies are created, and they move on to infect many cells. Hanging around in the body for long periods, they cause chronic or recurrent disease and also ensure their own long-term survival—it does them no good to kill off a host quickly. Over the long haul, hepatitis can alter the behavior of cells and cause them to become cancerous.

# Hepatitis B

## CORDYCEPS

Hepatitis B can cause cirrhosis of the liver, a very serious condition. People with advanced hepatitis and cirrhosis tend to develop ascites, in which free fluid accumulates in the abdomen, as well as generalized edema, in which too much fluid accumulates in the tissues themselves, causing swelling. Normally, albumin, a protein manufactured in the liver, acts as a water trap and prevents ascites and edema from occurring. When a diseased liver can't manufacture enough albumin, however, the result may be puffiness, particularly in the ankles, abdomen, and face. If albumin levels begin to rise, it means that some liver cells are still active and recovery may occur—which unfortunately rarely happens in hepatitis-induced cirrhosis. Instead, doctors try to prevent further damage by cautioning patients to avoid alcohol and drugs that might destroy what's left of the liver.

Small but impressive studies on hepatitis B-induced cirrhosis and glyconutrients have been conducted in China. In a 1986 open-label cordyceps study, researchers treated twenty-two very sick patients with cirrhosis from hepatitis B for three months.[2] Their blood work and symptoms improved: ascites resolved in 70 percent of the patients, and the other 30 percent showed improvement. In addition, immunoglobulins decreased, another important sign of recovery.

Other studies back up cordyceps's efficacy against hepatitis and cirrhosis. In one placebo-controlled study at the Shanghai Academy of TCM and Pharmacology, scientists found that cordyceps normalized immune functioning and reduced cirrhosis symptoms in hepatitis B patients.[3] And in a 1990 trial at the Shanxi Liver Diseases Research Co-operation Group in China, thirty-three patients with chronic hepatitis B took cordyceps daily for three months. At the end of the study, the researchers calculated a significant increase in albumin as well as a significant *decrease* in a key immunoglobulin called gammaglobulin (an antibody that tends to increase in people with hepatitis).[4]

Cordyceps mushrooms may help the liver recover by boosting

adenosine triphosphate, better known as ATP, the energy stored in the cells for immediate use. In one study, ATP levels in the liver rose considerably in mice fed cordyceps extracts for seven days, compared with controls.[5] The increase, however, dropped back to pre-treatment levels after the glyconutrients were discontinued for a week. In a rat study, researchers found that when reishi mushroom extracts were given together with the amino acid glutathione, a potent antioxidant, the damage done by chemically induced hepatitis was reduced far more effectively than with either substance alone.[6]

*Suggested Use:* Always get your doctor's approval before adding glyconutrients to your medical treatment. Try 3 to 9 grams of cordyceps extracts or Cs-4 daily, in divided doses. People with edema and ascites in some cases receive additional benefit with the higher doses of 6 to 9 grams daily, in divided doses. But start with 500 milligrams daily and build up gradually.

Until researchers conduct human studies, we won't know if reishi (with or without glutathione) is an effective treatment for people with hepatitis. However, reishi extracts are good immune-system boosters, at 1 to 9 grams daily, in divided doses.

## REISHI AND MAITAKE

In hepatitis B patients, reishi and maitake extracts lower liver enzymes, enhancing the liver's detoxifying capabilities.[7, 8] In a study of thirty-two patients with chronic hepatitis B discussed in a review article, Chinese researchers found that about two-thirds of the group given maitake extracts had significant drops in a liver enzyme called alanine transferase, which is elevated in the disease; only about half of the controls, who received standard drug treatment, experienced reductions in the enzyme.[9] In addition, the maitake group experienced a significantly higher rate of remission.

*Suggested Use:* Always get your doctor's approval before adding glyconutrients to your medical treatment. Try 3 to 9 grams of maitake extract daily, in divided doses. Maitake D-fraction: 0.5 to 1.0 milligram per kilogram of body weight daily, in three divided doses. To find your weight in kilograms, multiply your weight in

pounds by 0.45. For example, a 120-pound woman weighs 54 kilos and would take 27 to 54 milligrams of maitake D-fraction per
day. Reishi extract: 3 to 9 grams of reishi extract daily, in divided
doses. Caution: Consult your doctor before taking reishi if you
have a bleeding disorder or are taking blood thinners. If you have
edema or ascites, the higher doses of glyconutrients, in some
cases, are more effective—but start out slowly and increase the
dosage gradually. If you combine two glyconutrients, cut the
dose for each by half; if you combine three, cut the dose for each
by two-thirds, and so on.

## Hepatitis C and Liver Cancer

An extract from the shiitake mushroom, active hexose correlated
compound (AHCC), has been shown to increase survival time
and quality of life of patients with liver cancer caused by hepatitis C. Japanese researchers found that in patients with hepatitis-
induced cancer, key blood markers that indicate liver damage
fell, while both white blood cell and red blood cell counts rose,
when patients were administered 3 grams of the glyconutrient,
as compared with controls, whose blood work did not improve.[10]
Glyconutrient patients also reported an increase in appetite. Although survival, blood work, and quality of life improved in the
AHCC-treated group more than in the controls, tumor recurrence did *not* decline.

   *Suggested Use:* Always get your doctor's approval before adding
glyconutrients to your medical treatment. Three to four grams of
AHCC daily, in divided doses.

## HIV

Viruses that infect humans have an affinity for certain kinds of
cells and tissues and not for others because for a virus to enter a
cell, it first must attach itself to a cell membrane. Different
viruses attach to different cells. The HIV virus has an affinity for

the CD4 cells, also called helper T cells, which the virus slowly destroys. Here's where saccharides come in: The presence of essential saccharides on the skin or in the diet can often confuse a virus at critical points in its acquisition of its victim's cell—and the virus can't secure a foothold. Poor diet and illness can lead to essential-saccharide deficiencies that leave a chink in our defenses, making us more susceptible to viruses, which then can gain the upper hand.

A glycoprotein called gp120—which looks like knobs on the HIV virus—must be present for the HIV virus to attach itself properly to its victim's cells. Indefatigable virologist Don Francis, one of the few heroes in *And the Band Played On*, Randy Shilts's book on how politics helped launch the AIDS epidemic,[11] has developed an AIDS vaccine called gp120 with the biomedical company Genentech.[12] The vaccine, in Phase III human trials, manipulates glycoprotein 120, purportedly rendering HIV unable to infect. Would taking glyconutrients help prevent you from contracting HIV? Until studies are done, we won't know if they're helpful. But we do know that glyconutrients improve immune function. To boost overall immunity, see my recommendation below.

Glyconutrients have been found to increase the potency of traditional AIDS drugs in humans. In one study, for instance, intravenous lentinan, an extract from the shiitake mushroom, increased helper T cell counts in AIDS patients by an average of 142 when given in combination with the AIDS drug ddI; controls who received only ddI experienced a *decrease* of helper Ts.[13] Patients received 1 to 10 milligrams of lentinan once or twice a week for eight to twelve weeks. Another controlled lentinan-ddI study, using 2 milligrams of intravenous lentinan for twenty-four to eighty weeks, confirmed these findings.[14] In addition, there have been anecdotal reports that maitake D-fraction extract is effective against Kaposi's sarcoma, a skin cancer common in AIDS patients that's identified by telltale bluish-red nodules.[15]

All the news on the glyconutrient front, however, is not as encouraging. In a 1996 double-blind acemannan study in advanced HIV disease, patients who received the saccharide didn't fare any better than those taking a placebo.[16] One reason for the finding may be that the patients were so ill. Glyconutrient supplementation, like most treatments, seems to be more effective if begun earlier in the disease process.

*Suggested Use:* Research studies on HIV and saccharides have been small, so no firm conclusions about saccharides' effects on the HIV virus can be drawn. But the evidence so far is encouraging. To adults with HIV and other serious immune-system disorders, I recommend taking a variety of glyconutrients to support the immune system. Start with one at a time, and build up gradually. Maitake D-fraction: 7 to 10 milligrams per day. Cordyceps extracts or Cs-4: 1 gram a day, in divided doses. Reishi extracts: 1 gram a day in divided doses. Caution: If you have a bleeding disorder or take aspirin or other blood thinners, consult your doctor before adding cordyceps or reishi extracts. Stabilized powdered *Aloe vera:* 250 milligrams two times a day. Rice or yeast bran: Follow manufacturer's recommendations or your doctor's advice. Read labels carefully: To enhance flavor, some manufacturers add sweetener and other additives to brans. Also consider adding shiitake, oyster, and maitake mushrooms to your diet.

Oral lentinan: 12.5 milligrams twice a day, if you are taking only lentinan. If you are taking other glyconutrients, cut the oral lentinan dose in half.

Lentinan is usually more effective by injection than orally. Injectable lentinan is available by prescription only and must be administered to adults under a physician's supervision. Serious side effects have occurred with IV lentinan, including fever, chills, back and leg pain, elevated liver enzymes, and anaphylaxis—a serious and potentially fatal allergic reaction. Do not use injectable lentinan if you take the prescription anti-inflammatory drug indomethacin (Indocin). See chapter 3 for more information. Lentinan doses are calculated by a physician according to the patient's weight and health status. Children should not take injectable lentinan.

Feline leukemia virus shares similarities with the HIV retrovirus, and acemannan from aloe has also been shown to improve the survival rates and the health of cats infected with it.[17] In a test-tube study in which the aloe extract was used in conjunction with the AIDS drug AZT, the glyconutrient acted synergistically with the drug to hinder the replication of the HIV virus.[18]

## Infections in Immunocompromised Patients

In the early 1980s, when I was working as a young doctor at a rural Catholic hospital in Southern Cameroons, Africa, we admitted a twenty-year-old man I'll call Kenjo. He had been stabbed in the abdomen, a rare occurrence in that mountainous region. We heard two versions of how his injury came about: one was that he had been caught stealing; the other was that he had been caught with another man's wife. However the injury occurred, Kenjo was in shock and bleeding internally. His spleen had ruptured, and the only treatment for a ruptured spleen is surgical removal. Individuals with no spleen are at high risk of death from bacterial infection, but we had no choice. We gave him a blood transfusion and started him on penicillin to protect him from deadly bacterial infections that could result. He rapidly recovered, returning to his boisterous self within a few days, flirting with the nurses.

We were planning his discharge when suddenly he took ill with a strep infection. He developed a fever and huge bloody patches on his skin called purpurae and quickly lapsed into shock and coma. Though we took rapid action to arrest the infection, the young man was dead in less than two hours. In most people, strep throat is a nuisance. For those without spleens, it can be a deadly infection, comparable with—or more lethal than—the Ebola virus in the sudden and dramatic way in which it can take a life.

Not having a spleen is not as uncommon in this country as you might expect. Car accidents cause many ruptured spleens every year. And people who suffer from sickle cell disease often lose their spleens to the disease in the first two decades of life. The blood supply is simply lost to different small portions of the spleen, and over time the spleen often dies from lack of oxygen.

As a result, sickle cell patients have generally diminished immunity. That is one reason those with the disease take penicillin daily.

Unfortunately, as more germs are becoming resistant to penicillin, doctors are turning to less-safe, broad-spectrum antibiotics to treat patients. Glyconutrients may be of help here, too, because they boost the workings of the immune system, including increasing the production of the enzyme glutathione synthetase in cells, which in turn produces the powerful antioxidant glutathione.[19, 20, 21] Glyconutrients do not interfere with the effectiveness of antibiotics—unless the directions require that you take the antibiotics on an empty stomach—because unlike antibiotics, glyconutrients do not kill bacteria. Instead, glyconutrients empower the immune system to do its own killing. We know that glutathione levels are low in those with sickle cell anemia, and this may contribute to patients' susceptibility to painful sickle-cell crises. More research on glyconutrients and sickle-cell disease is indicated, as treatment of patients in distress usually means pulling out the big guns: narcotic painkillers, blood transfusions, bone-marrow transplants, and intensive-care stays.

*Suggested Use:* For immunocompromised adults, I recommend supplementation with a variety of glyconutrients or with a glyconutrient complex that contains several of the eight essential saccharides. (See the resources chapter for more information.) If you prefer to try glyconutrients individually, start with one at a time and build up gradually. Maitake D-fraction: 7 to 10 milligrams per day. Cordyceps extract or Cs-4: 1 gram a day, in divided doses. Reishi extracts: 1 gram a day in divided doses. Caution: If you have blood-coagulation problems or are taking aspirin or other blood thinners, consult your doctor before adding Cs-4, cordyceps, or reishi extracts, as these glyconutrients can cause bleeding problems. Stabilized powdered *Aloe vera*: 250 milligrams once a day. Rice bran: Follow manufacturer's recommendations. Read labels carefully: To enhance flavor, some manufacturers add sweetener. Yeast beta-glucans: 20 to 40 milligrams once a day. Also consider adding shiitake, oyster, and maitake mushrooms to your diet. Polysaccharide K: Although human studies haven't been conducted using this glyconutrient to treat opportunistic infections, we know that the glyconutrient enhances immune function at 1-6 grams a day, in divided doses. Start out slowly, and build gradually. Occasionally, polysaccharide K causes a benign darkening of the fingernails. Children under 12 should not take polysaccharide K.

Animal experiments using glyconutrients on mice whose spleens have been surgically removed offer new reason for hope for human patients. In one study, the incidence of infection increased and survival rate decreased when mice were inoculated with the strep bacterium that causes pneumonia (the most common cause of bacterial pneumonia). Immunity of the mice was also compromised by strep, as well as by *E. coli* and *Pseudomonas aeruginosa* (which can cause a variety of infections in compromised individuals), when the mice were implanted with tumors, but was restored in mice fed polysaccharide K from the mushroom *Coriolus versicolor.*[22] Indeed, in another study, researchers were surprised to find that the survival rates of tumor-bearing mice and rats with surgically removed spleens were actually *better* than those of tumor-bearing rodents with intact spleens when both groups were administered glyconutrients.[23]

Other experiments using polysaccharide K to fight *Pseudomonas aeruginosa* bacteria in mice with tumors have been equally encouraging.[24] An opportunistic bacterium because it tends to infect premature infants and the immunosuppressed, *P. aeruginosa* can trigger life-threatening wound infections in burn patients and chronic lung infections in those with cystic fibrosis. But in several in vitro studies at University of British Columbia, University of Texas, and elsewhere, saccharides have inhibited the attachment of that bacterium to the tissues and respiratory tract.[25, 26, 27]

## Averting Antibiotic Damage in Immune-Suppressed Patients

When broad-spectrum antibiotics are called for to treat bacterial infections, adding glyconutrients can protect kidneys from the damage that antibiotics sometimes cause, particularly in immune-compromised or older adults. In a controlled study with cordyceps mushrooms, twenty-one elderly patients with severe infections, including bronchitis and pneumonia, were divided into two groups. For six days, both groups received injections of the antibiotic amikacin, which can lead to renal toxicity. But only one group got cordyceps; the control group got a placebo. The researchers found that the cordyceps/amikacin group experienced significantly less kidney damage than the amikacin-only group. This means that the cordyceps protected the kidneys from antibiotic-induced damage.[28]

*Suggested Use:* 3 to 6 grams of cordyceps extract or Cs-4 daily, in divided doses. Caution: If you have a bleeding disorder or are taking a blood-thinner, including aspirin, consult your doctor before adding cordyceps or Cs-4.

In the immunocompromised, glyconutrients can be helpful in treating serious bacterial and viral infections. Although glyconutrients should not be used in lieu of current treatment protocols, studies do indicate that glyconutrients may be valuable, synergistic accompaniments to today's antibiotics and antivirals in treating hepatitis, HIV, and opportunistic infections.

# PART III

# TURN BACK THE CLOCK

"If I'd known I was gonna live this long, I'd
have taken better care of myself."
—*Eubie Blake, musician, at age 100*

## Chapter 13

# Glyconutrients as Preventive Self-Care

*How glyconutrients help slow down aging; increase
endurance, sexual function, and fertility; reduce body fat
and build muscle; and prevent altitude sickness.*

**W**hile trying to pick out an appropriate quotation to start this
section of the book, I was struck with just how many quotations
there are about aging. Some are old-fashioned funny ("I don't
generally feel anything until noon, then it's time for my nap,"
from Bob Hope); others are jaded ("I'm not getting older, I'm
getting bitter," decrees the slogan emblazoned on a T-shirt popular in Greenwich Village). Then come the resigned ("The older
you get, the better you used to be," uttered by NBA Hall of
Famer Connie Hawkins), and the buoyant (Norman Vincent
Peale's "Live your life and forget your age"). Victor Hugo's
"Forty is the old age of youth. Fifty is the youth of old age" is re-
flective, while T. S. Eliot's is wry: "The years between fifty and seventy are the hardest. You are always being asked to do things,
and yet you are not decrepit enough to turn them down." Then
there's Tina Turner's defiant, "I will never give in to old age until

I become old. And I'm not old yet!" One of my personal fa-
vorites, "He is so old that his blood type was discontinued," is
courtesy of comedian Bill Dana.

No one I know looks forward to growing old, but as a wise person once said, it beats the alternative. As we age our bodies begin
to lose the fight against time. Our immune systems become less
accurate and less active against bacteria, viruses, and cancer, and
we become more prone to develop autoimmune diseases. We lose
lean tissue, which makes up our organs, muscle, connective tissue, and bone. This degeneration leads to injuries, slow healing,
and osteoporosis. At the same time, the percentage of body fat increases. These physical changes correlate very well with the loss of
immune function and progression to age-related disability.

Nutritional studies tell us that the foods we eat play a particularly crucial role in graceful aging. The immune systems of well-
nourished older individuals tend to be nearly as robust as those of
people younger than forty, but researchers at Pennsylvania State
University postulate that nutritional status is often overlooked in
evaluating the immune systems of the old versus those of the young.
In a study that examined the immune status of well-nourished
older women sixty-two to eighty-eight years of age versus young
women twenty to forty, scientists reported no significant differences between most immune markers in the two age groups.[1]
Contrast their finding with that of scientists at Nagasaki University
School of Medicine in Japan, who uncovered significant depressed immune systems in the malnourished elderly.[2]

## Slowing Down Aging:
## Human and Animal Studies

Even with good nutrition and exercise we continue to age, albeit
at a slower pace. But glyconutrients offer hope that the slide can
be slowed even more—and in some cases reversed. How? Perhaps the biggest single factor in aging is free-radical damage. Superoxide dismutase (SOD) is a blood enzyme that destroys free
radicals. As people age, SOD levels tend to decrease; when SOD

is low, the level of free radicals is high. In several studies, the administration of 3 grams of the cordyceps mushroom extract Cs-4 for three months to elderly people with weakness and loss of strength resulted in significantly higher enzyme levels and fewer free radicals.[3] Cs-4 also lowered the levels of a blood marker called plasma malondialdehyde (MDA), which measures a free radical called lipoperoxide. In fact, researchers found that the lowered MDA levels and raised SOD levels in elderly patients after Cs-4 treatment *rivaled levels seen in young adults.* Chinese researchers replicated these impressive findings in a subsequent trial of elderly patients with senility.[4]

But it's not just the blood markers that improved: the patients felt better. Patients in the latter study, for instance, also reported a decrease in dizziness, chills, urinating at night, and ringing in the ears. In animals, other mushrooms have been proved efficacious as well in restoring youthful immune vigor and immune markers. A study conducted at Beijing Medical University in China found that when old mice were administered polysaccharides from the reishi mushroom, their immune function perked up to the point that levels of key immune markers in the spleen matched or surpassed those of young mice.[5]

*Suggested Use:* In China and Japan, cordyceps and reishi mushrooms are used to restore vigor and improve endurance. (For more information, see Building Endurance section, below.) Do not take cordyceps, Cs-4, or reishi extracts if you're on a blood thinner or have a bleeding disorder unless directed by a physician. Start out slowly with one glyconutrient at a time and increase dosage gradually. Cordyceps: 1 to 6 grams daily, in divided doses. Reishi: 1 to 6 grams daily, in divided doses. If you take both glyconutrients, cut the dose for each by half.

## Building Endurance

Rebecca is a fifty-seven-year-old grandmother who works as a housekeeper at one of the hospitals with which I'm affiliated. Over the past nine years we have become friends. Until two years ago, her health had been good and stable and her health complaints minor—the occasional flu and seasonal allergies. About a year and a half ago, however, her health started to deteriorate; she complained of being "wiped out"—exhausted. Her doctor, she said, had run a number of tests to ascertain what was wrong. Her heart was normal except for mildly elevated blood pressure; her thyroid was normal, and she wasn't anemic. Other blood work all came back negative. As she had already been through menopause, her symptoms couldn't be attributed to change of life. She told me she was having difficulty keeping up with the demands of her job, with its eight- to twelve-hour shifts, and she was worried. I briefly considered that Rebecca might have chronic fatigue syndrome (CFS), but she didn't have the sore throat, swollen glands, and memory problems of CFS patients—and most CFS patients have low blood pressure, not high.

A few months passed and Rebecca had not improved. I suggested that she might trying supplementing her diet with glyconutrients. She did, taking a blend of stabilized, powdered *Aloe vera* and gum sugars, 500 milligrams once daily, as well 2 grams of cordyceps extract daily, in divided doses. (See the resources chapter for more information.) Two weeks later she reported a subtle but definite improvement in her energy. She continued to improve over the next several months, until she felt well. In fact, she told me she feels better now than she felt before she became ill. She has continued on a maintenance intake of glyconutrients, halving her daily dose.

No one can say for sure whether Rebecca's health improved because she took glyconutrients. If she had an illness we could not diagnose, it could have run its course naturally, or her improvement could have been due to a placebo effect—in other words, her expectations of getting well, not the glyconutrients, helped her body recover. However, other anecdotal evidence and animal studies have borne out that glyconutrients, particularly cordyceps and reishi extracts, help build endurance. As discussed in chapter 1, Chinese swimmers attributed their success in breaking nine world records in the 1993 Chinese National Games to cordyceps mushrooms. A year later Chinese researchers found that the reishi mushroom makes *mice* better swimmers. In fact, mice administered reishi extract for seven days before a swimming endurance test experienced a 27 to 52 percent increase in swimming time—depending upon the reishi dose, with the higher doses being more effective.[6]

Humans receive added resilience from reishi as well: in a Chinese study that examined reishi's effects on high-altitude sickness, which causes, among other symptoms, headaches and vomiting, 900 male soldiers took 1 gram of reishi extract daily in two divided doses for six days while driving in the cold to an elevation of more than 15,000 feet.[7] Most of the soldiers— 82 percent—completed the journey without headaches; 94 percent completed the experiment without vomiting. The data were compared with earlier figures from the Chinese Academy of Army Medicine in Beijing, which held that unless pretreated with medication, most of the soldiers traveling to that elevation experienced symptoms of high-altitude sickness, including headaches and vomiting.

*Suggested Use:* Reishi and cordyceps extracts have become an integral part of the diets of many athletes. Take 1 to 6 grams daily of reishi, cordyceps, or Cs-4 extracts, in divided amounts. If you decide to use both mushrooms, halve the dose for each. Caution: Do not take reishi, cordyceps, or the cordyceps extract Cs-4 if you take a blood thinner or have a bleeding disorder unless under a doctor's care.

## Sexual Desire, Function, and Fertility

Before there was Viagra, there was the cordyceps mushroom, long used in traditional Chinese medicine to treat both erectile dysfunction and low libido. Cordyceps appears to revitalize tissues structurally and functionally, increasing estrogen and testosterone production, whereas Viagra causes dilation of the penile arteries and increased blood flow to the penis. Viagra treats erectile dysfunction only—it doesn't affect libido per se— and its effects are transient. Viagra, unlike cordyceps, often can't be taken by people with heart disease. One drawback of cordyceps, however, is that it takes anywhere from a week to a few months to work; Viagra informs the user within an hour that it's operational.

In 1995, Chinese researchers conducted a forty-day trial of 256 elderly male and female patients complaining of diminished libido and impotence.[8] Some 64 percent of cordyceps patients, who took 3 grams of the glyconutrient daily, reported subjective improvement in libido and function, versus 23 percent of placebo patients. The scientists also found that those taking cordyceps were producing more sex hormones. In another trial, after twenty-two male patients with complete impotence were treated with 3 grams of Cs-4 for eight weeks, more than one-third were capable of sexual intercourse.[9] In addition, sperm counts rose 33 percent, malformed sperm decreased by 29 percent, and sperm survival rate increased from 29 percent pretreatment to an impressive 52 percent posttreatment.

Animal studies have confirmed the sperm-count increases: after male rabbits were treated with a cordyceps extract for three months, their sperm count tripled compared to controls, the number of defective sperm was reduced, and survival time increased.[10] The glyconutrient-exposed rabbits also had a 30 percent increase in testicle size, and the super-testicles were normal in structure. Along the same lines, premature female mice administered cordyceps infusions for six days experienced a 43 percent increase in uterine weight.[11]

*Suggested Use:* Consult your doctor before trying cordyceps to treat sexual desire or fertility problems or menopausal symptoms. If you are already taking estrogen, testosterone, or DHEA (an adrenal hormone that produces estrogen and testosterone), do *not* add cordyceps unless under a doctor's care; your doctor may need to lower your estrogen or testosterone dose. Cordyceps causes an increase in testosterone and estrogen production, which may be problematic or even contraindicated in certain people, including those who have estrogen- or testosterone-sensitive cancers or have a family history of cancer, particularly breast, uterine, ovarian, cervical, prostate, and testicular. Once your doctor gives the okay, I recommend 1 to 3 grams of cordyceps extract or Cs-4, in divided doses.

## Staving Off Fat, Preserving Muscle

Body fat is increasing in the young and old alike in the United States because of the prevalent high-sugar, high-fat diet and couch-potato lifestyle. Obesity, which technically means being 20 percent or more over ideal weight, is a serious problem and getting worse. A third of Americans are obese, up about 8 percent from twenty years ago.[12] And children, especially, are at risk: in the past twenty years the number of obese children has doubled.

Serious health problems that may result from excess weight, combined with the cultural stigma tied to being overweight, have fed the multibillion-dollar diet business, as well as the exercise and pharmaceutical industries. Most of these diets and weight-loss drugs, however, have produced disappointing or short-lived results, and some drugs, like the diet pill combo of fenfluramine and phentermine—nicknamed fen-phen—have been found to be dangerous, resulting in heart-valve damage in some cases.

So it seems an oxymoron to think that the eight essential sugars will help people lose weight. After all, we're continually being bombarded with messages about the evils of excessive sugar consumption. Sugars that are not used up, for instance, are converted into fat and stored in unattractive deposits around the body. Too much sugar in the diet can lead to diabetes and heart disease. But the daily quantity needed in a healthy diet of these eight essential sugars is quite small—a half to a whole teaspoon a day, for most people. Many controlled, double-blind studies on obesity and glyconutrients have been conducted on animals and people, with encouraging results.

Researchers at the Koseikai Clinic in Tokyo modified the diets of thirty overweight patients by giving them each powdered maitake mushrooms equivalent to 200 grams daily of fresh mushrooms for two months.[13] (Two hundred grams is 0.44 of a pound, a little less than a half-pound. Because the whole mushroom is not concentrated like extracts, you can take more.) Otherwise, researchers didn't change the patients' eating habits. All the patients lost significant weight, ranging from 11 to 26 pounds. Maitake mushrooms can cause cramping, loose stools, or diarrhea. If you experience any of these reactions, reduce your mushroom intake until the problems resolve, to prevent dehydration and water-weight loss.

Glyconutrients not only help you lose weight, they help you lose the right kind of weight. In most diets you lose muscle as well as fat, and weight loss is not an accurate indication of fat loss. Your bathroom scale can't tell you if you've lost fat or fat-free mass—fancy words for lean tissue, which includes muscle, bone, connective tissue, and internal organs. Just as loss of lean tissue is one of the markers of aging and decreased immune functioning, loss of fat is associated with improved health and independence. Significant lean-tissue loss results in a starvation state in which the body actually cannibalizes itself, burning away muscle, heart, liver, and other organs while sparing fat. Anorexia is an extreme example of this phenomenon, which can lead to death.

Using a DEXA scan, which measures the percentages of body fat and lean tissue (it can also measure bone density), researchers studied 136 overweight people.[14] One group was placed on weight-loss drugs and a recommended diet and exercise plan in step with their goal weight. Another group was placed on a weight-loss drug, a diet and exercise plan, as well as *Aloe vera* extracts and phytochemicals (freeze-dried fruits and vegetables). The third group was placed on a diet and exercise plan, *Aloe vera*, and phytochemical supplements—but no weight-loss drugs.

DEXA scans were conducted at the beginning and at the end of the sixty-day study. The scientists found that those on glyconutrients and phytochemicals *consistently gained lean tissue and lost fat to a more significant degree than those on drugs alone.* Specifically, the drug-only group lost 0.8 percent of body fat, as compared to 4 percent in the drug/supplement group and 3.5 percent in the supplement-only group. The drug-only group lost 2.9 pounds of muscle, whereas the drug/supplement group *gained* 2.4 pounds of muscle and the supplement-only group *gained* nearly 4 pounds of muscle. The two groups that took weight-loss drugs each lost about 8.5 pounds, whereas the supplement group lost only 4 pounds—but keep in mind that the supplement-only group gained more muscle than the other two groups, and muscle is denser and weighs more than fat. That's why muscular people may weigh more but look slimmer than their flabby counterparts.

How much weight loss was attributable to the *Aloe vera* and how much to phytochemicals in this study isn't known, though animal studies confirm that glyconutrients alone aid in weight loss. In one study, scientists at the Kobe Pharmaceutical University in Japan fed ten young rats with high cholesterol and triglyceride levels a high-fat diet laced with maitake powder.[15] The ten controls received the high-fat feed without the mushroom powder. After twenty-four days, while both groups had put on weight, the controls had put on considerably more. As an added maitake bonus, the maitake rats registered significantly lower triglyceride and total cholesterol levels than the controls at the end of the study.

*Suggested Use:* 250 milligrams of stabilized powdered *Aloe vera* extract, one to three times daily. Maitake extract: 3 to 6 grams daily, in divided doses, or add up to a half-pound of cooked maitake mushrooms to your diet daily. If you experience cramping or diarrhea, cut back on your intake.

## WEIGHT LOSS: A PATIENT'S SUCCESS

Stephen wanted to lose weight. He's thirty-seven years old, big-boned, and at 5 feet 7 inches tall weighs 230. A good friend, he knew about my interest in glyconutrients. "Would glyconutrients help me take off weight?" he wanted to know. My first reaction was to give him a dose of reality: "Unfortunately, there's no magic in weight loss," I told him. Anybody who successfully takes off and keeps off weight has made a permanent commitment to exercise and eating healthfully. Weight loss is never easy, and no pill or food can make it effortless.

By exercising and eating sensibly, Stephen had lost weight before, but eventually returned to his old eating habits and sedentary lifestyle. This time, he promised things would be different. Encouraged by his wife, he eliminated the junk food he craved and committed to exercise. Since Stephen hates going to the gym—he says he would sooner mow the lawn than exhibit himself in a gym—he started walking three to five miles three times a week.

In addition, Stephen added, on my recommendation, 3 grams of the glyconutrient chitosan, a half-hour before lunch and dinner. Like the polysaccharide chitin, chitosan is found in the shells of crustaceans, including shrimp, krill, and crabs. Chitin modified by acid and alkali becomes chitosan, which binds fat in the digestive tract, preventing its digestion and absorption. I cautioned him that since he was using chitosan, he should also supplement with a good multivitamin a half-hour *after* lunch and dinner because fat-soluble vitamins might also be lost with the chitosan. In addition, I advised him to add shiitake and maitake mushrooms to his diet because they contain immune-boosting glyconutrients. Stephen also added 1 to 2 grams of cordyceps extracts, in divided amounts daily.

Unlike his previous weight-loss attempts, Stephen remarked that he wasn't experiencing hunger pangs as frequently this time around. In addition, he noticed he had more stamina and an increased sense of well-being. (Others who've used glyconutrients to lose weight have told me that their cravings diminished and their stamina increased as well.) In the first month, Stephen lost 5 pounds. Five months later, he had lost another 35. He stabilized at 190 and has kept the weight off for three years.

*Suggested Use:* 1 to 3 grams of chitosan a half-hour before meals. Caution: Do *not* take chitosan if you're allergic to shellfish, as the glyconutrient is derived from shellfish. If you add chitosan to your diet, make sure you take a multivitamin a half-hour after meals, once or twice daily. Cordyceps extracts or Cs-4 may also help boost immunity: 1 to 3 grams in divided doses, in this case a half-hour *after* meals. Consider adding cooked mushrooms to your diet as well.

# Sun Damage

The sun emits a large spectrum of radiation, including visible light, by which you may be reading this page. Infrared and ultraviolet rays are invisible parts of the spectrum, and part of the ultraviolet spectrum is responsible for activating vitamin D in our skin. While we require a certain minimum of exposure to sunlight to activate vitamin D, portions of the ultraviolet spectrum called UVA and UVB can cause severe damage to the skin if we're overexposed. Traditional sunscreens are designed to prevent the penetration of UVB, the ultraviolet radiation that causes fair skin to burn and darker skins to bronze when exposed to sun. Some of the newer formulations prevent the more insidious UVA as well.

Both kinds of radiation accelerate the aging of the skin by destroying collagen, which leads to leathery skin, broken blood vessels, blotchy pigmentation, sagging, wrinkles, and sometimes skin cancer. Even if you use a sunscreen with a high SPF number, the protection is incomplete, so it's still a bad idea to get too much sun no matter what you slather on your skin. (Zinc oxide—the gooey, white ointment usually reserved for the nose—does block out all UVA and UVB radiation, however.)

Sunscreen does nothing to reverse skin damage once the damage is done. And if the damage is severe enough, it may induce suppression of the Langerhans cells, located in the skin's epidermis, the outer layer of skin. This suppression results in reduced immunity in the skin, which may precede malignancy. Langerhans cells, a kind of macrophage, coordinate the actions of the immune system, orchestrating skin healing. *Aloe vera* gel has been shown to prevent the suppression of these cells in mice, thereby preventing ultraviolet-induced immune suppression in the skin.[16] In animals, aloe's ability to prevent skin damage from the sun and from radiation treatment for cancer has been documented extensively.[17]

In 1994, a research team at M.D. Anderson Cancer Center in Houston, Texas, found that mice exposed to UVB showed diminished immune response, with up to 90 percent less macrophage activity than in controls. Exposure to UVB can suppress immunity not only at the skin level but also throughout the body. Applying aloe gel to the skin within twenty-four hours after exposure to ultraviolet light restored Langerhans cells and immune functioning both locally and systemically.[18] M.D. Anderson scientists also reported that ordinary skin cells exposed to ultraviolet rays showed a decreased immune response, but aloe extracts restored the immune system response to normal.[19]

*Suggested Use:* Because only animal studies have been done on aloe's ability to prevent sun damage, scientists don't know if aloe will prevent sun damage in humans. However, studies have shown that topical application of stabilized *Aloe vera* speeds up healing in wounds and burns (see chapter 8), so it's a reasonable hypothesis that aloe will accelerate healing from sunburn. Before going into the sun, apply sun block. If you stay out too long, try stabilized aloe gel immediately *after* sun exposure. When applying *Aloe vera* for the first time, dab a little on an inconspicuous spot on your leg or arm and wait twenty-four hours to see if you develop an allergic reaction. If skin becomes red and itchy or you develop hives, discontinue use.

## Osteoporosis

By boosting estrogen levels, cordyceps mushrooms may help prevent osteoporosis, common in women after menopause. Although no formal human studies have been undertaken, other sugars have already been found to prevent bone loss in animals, including lactose (composed of glucose and galactose), lactulose (a synthetic sugar used to treat patients with advanced cirrhosis), and maltitol (from the malt sugar maltose, it's absorbed slowly and is used in sugar-free candy, gum, and chocolate in Europe).[20]

New findings indicate that a disaccharide (two sugars) of glucose called trehalose prevents osteoporosis in mice. In one study, scientists removed the ovaries from mice; one group received placebo and the other, trehalose.[21] Four weeks later, scientists reported that in the trehalose animals, the calcium and phosphorus content as well as the bone weight of the thighbones were significantly higher than those of the control mice. What's also significant is that the trehalose did *not* increase the weight of the animals' uteruses—which would be expected if trehalose preserved bone by boosting estrogen levels. The authors of the study suggest that trehalose may have certain benefits over estrogen in treating osteoporosis, as the hormone has been implicated in some gynecological cancers.

These findings are particularly timely because trehalose is about to become a household name. The international distributor Cargill, in conjunction with the Japanese company Hayashibara, which developed the product, is scheduled to market the sweetener in the United States in soft drinks and other foods by the end of the year. The sugar is less sweet than table sugar—45 percent less sweet, to be exact. Trehalose has other properties besides taste and is already used both as a preservative for pharmaceutical products and as a moisture-retainer in cosmetics.

*Suggested Use:* Until human trials are conducted on trehalose and osteoporosis, scientists won't know whether the glyconutrient will prevent osteoporosis in people.

## Cataracts

Cataracts are the loss of transparency of the lens of the eye, and the incidence increases as we age. Exposure to sunlight, prolonged use of steroids, certain viral illnesses, and genetic predisposition are some of the other contributors. Interestingly, in one study researchers discovered that supplementing with galactose protected mice exposed to X-ray radiation from developing cataracts.[22] The researchers speculated that galactose, an essential saccharide ample in milk products, might act as a free-radical scavenger. In a follow-up study, scientists found that four months after X-ray exposure, about 50 percent of the galactose-fed group had mature cataracts, compared with 100 percent of the control group.[23]

*Suggested Use:* Studies have not been conducted to determine the effects of galactose on cataract development in humans, and, in any event, most people get plenty of galactose in their diets with dairy products. Once cataracts are fully formed, the only way to eliminate them is by surgery; no dietary changes can do that. If you have a family history of cataracts, eating your fair share of dairy products can't hurt—unless of course you have an allergy or milk intolerance. Other excellent sources of galactose are figs, grapes, peas, tomatoes, hazelnuts, beans, and pectin supplements.

Glyconutrients can help rejuvenate the immune systems of aging animals to resemble those of their friskier, younger counterparts. Glyconutrients stave off body fat, preserve lean tissue, improve stamina, prevent altitude sickness, and perk up sexual desire and functioning. These findings serve as compelling evidence that glyconutrients can help slow the aging process, and in some cases reverse it.

## Chapter 14

# Working with Memory, Insomnia, Anxiety, Depression, and ADHD

*Glyconutrients' effects on the brain and nervous system.*

**M**uch of the material covered so far in this book concerns the immune system. That's because it's relatively easy to study by analyzing the white blood cells present in a patient's blood sample. But examining the nervous system is another matter entirely, so the brain remains somewhat mysterious. Researchers cannot open up the intact brain of a living human being to satisfy our curiosity, so they employ indirect methods, using PET scans, MRIs, and postmortem studies, as well as studying other animals whose brains are extraordinarily similar to ours. Nature has a way of reusing successful organs, structures, and adaptations across species.

Saccharides play a significant role in the work of nerve tissue, especially during brain development.[1, 2] Galactolipids, composed of saccharides and fats, are found on the myelin sheaths on nerves, insulating the nerve fibers much like the plastic coating that covers electrical wires. Several studies have examined the role of galactolipids in nervous system function. In one, mice genetically engineered to be devoid of these myelin galactolipids developed severe tremors, paralysis, and poor formation of the myelin sheath and nerve fibers.[3]

Glycoproteins on nerve cell surfaces are receptors of molecules called neurotransmitters, including norepinephrine, dopamine, and serotonin. Disruption of these neurotransmitters and their glycoprotein receptors sets off a chain of biochemical events that results in abnormalities in our movements, thoughts, and feelings. In Parkinson's disease, for example, dopamine is depleted as the cells that produce it die off, resulting in tremors and rigidity; depressed and suicidal patients often register lower levels of serotonin.

The thrust of treating some neurological and psychiatric diseases centers on medications that *increase* the quantity or life span of these neurochemicals or that *block* their actions. Although these medications do treat the symptoms, they are fraught with side effects. Nutritional supplementation may hold more promise than current medications. Fatty-acid deficiencies, for instance, have been found in those with Parkinson's disease, Alzheimer's disease, multiple sclerosis, schizophrenia, depression, manicdepression, and attention deficit hyperactivity disorder (ADHD); studies using fish oil, which supplies the missing fats, have been encouraging.[4, 5, 6, 7, 8, 9, 10]

Animals studies (animals develop neurological disorders similar to our own) indicate that glyconutrients are also helpful in treating some of these illnesses. We know, for instance, that adding glyconutrients does affect the brain: in animal studies glyconutrients significantly curtail anxiety and alcohol's intoxicating effects—both acutely and long term. Animal studies also indicate that glyconutrients improve memory, increase intelligence, and decrease depression. (See the sections "Memory," "ADHD, Learning, Anxiety, and Behavior," and "Depression and Other Psychiatric Disorders," below.)

# Memory

Combining the dietary supplements L-carnitine, L-phosphatidyl serine, lecithin, borage oil, and flax oil has become a popular cocktail to improve memory. These nutrients are designed to support the lipid, or fatty, component of cell membranes. Cell membranes contain the receptors that receive signals from other brain cells; if the membranes are faulty, the brain will not function optimally, and memory, among other functions, can be adversely affected.

None of these aforementioned memory-cocktail nutrients contain glyconutrients, but essential saccharides do play crucial roles in cell membranes, which are made up of proteins, glycoproteins (molecules made of sugars and proteins), glycolipids (molecules made of sugars and fats), and phospholipids (the fats found in the cell membranes). So it's plausible that adding glyconutrients to the mix will further enhance memory in humans.

Already there's evidence that glyconutrients enhance memory in animals. In a 1999 study on rat brains, university researchers in Germany found that by blocking glycoprotein synthesis in the brain, memory formation did *not* occur. The scientists were evaluating what's called long-term potentiation (LTP), the quality that researchers look for when they study memory at the cellular level. LTP means that when nerve cells are repeatedly stimulated, the information becomes hard-wired; they remember the stimulus and facilitate it the next time around.[11] Other studies on rat brains indicate that the essential saccharide fucose and certain sugar compounds containing fucose improve memory formation.[12]

A study at the University of North Carolina School of Medicine showed the importance of glucosamine (a metabolic product of the essential saccharide N-acetylglucosamine) in learning.[13] After mice received glucosamine injections, half were returned to their cages and left alone, while the other half were given fifteen minutes' worth of avoidance-conditioning training, in which the mice were punished by electric shock for responding to some stimuli and rewarded with food for responding to others. Mice quickly learned what to avoid and what to touch. The researchers found that the trained mice incorporated 21 percent of the glucosamine into their brains, whereas the caged control groups incorporated only 12 percent.

*Suggested Use:* The animal studies are encouraging, but it's too early to say if supplementing with fucose, glucosamine, or other saccharides will help people as they've helped animals with learning and memory. Supplementing with glyconutrients, however, has been shown to improve immune functioning and decrease free radicals, and that in turn affects brain function. The brain uses about 20 percent of the body's total oxygen consumption—though it constitutes only one-fiftieth of the body's weight—and as free radicals need oxygen to survive, free-radical generation is heavily concentrated in the brain.[14] Unfortunately, compared with other tissues, the brain has a relatively poor supply of antioxidants. That combination makes the brain particularly susceptible to pathogens and toxins that generate free radicals. Adding a variety of cooked mushrooms or extracts (both are a good source of fucose) or supplementing with *Aloe vera*, arabinogalactans (gum sugars, another good source for fucose), or rice, oat, or barley brans can improve immune function. Follow manufacturer's instructions or your doctor's advice.

## Anxiety and Insomnia

In his book *Medicinal Mushrooms: An Exploration of Tradition, Healing, and Culture,* botanist Christopher Hobbs calls reishi the "calming" mushroom, particularly helpful for people with "anxiety, sleeplessness, or nervousness."[15] Animal studies support that claim.[16] In one study, rats given reishi extracts experienced significant increases in both REM sleep—the type of sleep in which rapid eye movement and dreaming occurs—and non-REM sleep, which constitutes the bulk, about 80 percent, of adult human sleep.[17]

*Suggested Use:* Although human studies have yet to be done, reishi has long been used in Japan and China as an antianxiety and sleep-promoting elixir. If you are suffering with moderate to severe anxiety or have a persistent sleep disorder, consult your physician. For occasional episodes of mild anxiety, try 1 to 9 grams of reishi extract daily with water, in divided doses. For occasional trouble falling asleep, take 1 to 3 grams of reishi extract with water an hour before bedtime. Do not take reishi extracts if you have a bleeding disorder or are taking a blood thinner unless your doctor gives you the okay.

## ADHD, Learning, Anxiety, and Behavior

Vince is ten years old and is the second-youngest of eight children. He was diagnosed with ADHD when he was four and a half years old. His is a severe case; he is in special education, is extraordinarily hyperactive, and has significant difficulty concentrating. He takes Ritalin, the most commonly used drug to treat ADHD, and clonidine, which is traditionally used to treat hypertension but has secured a niche as a second-line drug in ADHD. Because Ritalin suppresses appetite, Vince was eating little and losing weight. (Ritalin can also cause nausea and tremors, but Vince didn't experience those side effects.)

I decided to try him on a course of glyconutrients because I had heard anecdotal reports from other doctors of saccharides alleviating ADHD symptoms. One week after Vince started taking the glyconutrients (a combination of aloe and arabinogalactans, 500 milligrams, once a day; see the resources section for more information), his mother noted that his appetite had improved and that he seemed calmer. Three months later Vince finished the glyconutrient supply. Within two weeks he returned to baseline: his appetite was again poor and he was more fidgety. Once back on glyconutrients, he calmed down and resumed eating normally. There are no indications that long-term use of these natural supplements has any harmful side effects. Nevertheless, check with your doctor before starting your child on glyconutrients to avoid potential allergy problems.

Ritalin and another drug called Adderall are widely used—some experts would say overused—to treat ADHD, which affects 3 to 5 percent of children in the United States.[18] That so many kids and adults take drugs to function is a cause for concern. The fact remains, however, that children and adults with certain kinds of performance and attention problems are better able to concentrate and succeed at school and work when they take medication.

Factors such as pregnancy and delivery complications, family dysfunction, poverty, underlying mental and physical illnesses, and marital discord have all been suggested as causes or contributors to ADHD. Many experts also believe ADHD results from a defect in the neurochemical dopamine. It's hypothesized that either insufficient dopamine is produced or the glycoprotein receptors are insensitive and thereby not adequately stimulated by the dopamine that is generated.[19] How exactly stimulant medicines such as Ritalin work to increase attention and decrease hyperactivity isn't known, but they appear to cause changes in the way dopamine is metabolized. Ritalin may work by blocking dopamine's transporters, thereby increasing the amount of dopamine available for the neuroreceptors, which are glycoproteins.

Nutritional approaches to ADHD have been tried in the past. In the early 1970s, for instance, allergist Ben Feingold proposed that food additives, dyes, and natural salicylates (aspirin-like compounds) resulted in hyperactivity in susceptible children, and developed the Feingold Diet. This elimination diet fell out of favor a decade later, and double-blind studies have failed to uphold his theory.[20]

It's too early to tell if glyconutrients help definitively with ADHD, though anecdotal case histories like Vince's, as well as animal studies, suggest that they do. For instance, researchers at the College of Physicians and Surgeons at Columbia University in New York investigated the effects of malnutrition and environmental stimulation on the brain chemistry—including glycoprotein levels—of rat pups.[21] The pups were divided into four groups:

1. Well fed
2. Well fed and environmentally stimulated by presence of an adult female rat
3. Undernourished
4. Undernourished and environmentally stimulated by presence of an adult female rat

At the end of the three weeks the young rats received a battery of behavioral tests that evaluated attention, curiosity, learning speed, and anxiety. The researchers concluded that the brains of group 2 (the well-fed pups that were exposed to adult females) assimilated the *most* N-acetylneuraminic acid, one of the eight essential saccharides, particularly important for brain development and learning. In addition, this group was the most calm and learned a maze test the most quickly. This finding points to both diet and emotional stimulation playing a role in concentration and intelligence, which may prove important in treating ADHD and other learning disorders. These well-functioning rat pups also spent the most time checking out novel stimuli; in other words, they were more curious.

Coming in second in most categories were the well-fed pups without adult female rats. Not surprisingly, number 4, the poorly-nourished-without-an-adult-female group came in last in all categories. Interestingly, after the twenty-one-day trial, all the rats received the same diet and were housed in separate cages, yet the well-fed pups that had been in contact with adult females continued their superior performance. The other groups continued to perform at their previous levels as well. This indicates that both early environment and early nutrition have lasting effects on intelligence and behavior.

*Suggested Use:* Do not give glyconutrients to children with ADHD unless your doctor has approved. Then, only children two and up can take half of the manufacturer's recommended dose for aloe and arabinogalactans, or follow your doctor's instructions. Also consider adding cooked shiitake, maitake, and oyster mushrooms to your children's diets, as long as they aren't allergic to mushrooms.

# Depression and Other
# Psychiatric Disorders

Selective serotonin reuptake inhibitors—a type of antidepressant—
are among the best-selling drugs of all time. Now household
names, Prozac, Zoloft, and Paxil are the leaders of the pack, ele-
vating the moods of the clinically depressed. These antidepres-
sants work by preventing the reuptake of the neurotransmitter
serotonin, which means that the serotonin hangs around for a
longer period of time. That way, a higher concentration of serotonin is available to stimulate the dozen or so different kinds of
serotonin receptors, all of which are glycoproteins. An abnormality in the structure of at least some of these serotonin receptors is thought to be responsible for some cases of depression.

At Vanderbilt University in 1995, scientists showed that the
saccharides in these receptors play an important part in their
functioning.[22] That same year, Swiss researchers made a similar
observation.[23] And researchers at the University of Bonn in Germany found that suicidal psychiatric patients not only had low
blood levels of serotonin, their serotonin receptors were more
tightly bound to serotonin, suggesting a difference in the receptor structure.[24]

Since the neuroreceptors are glycoproteins, does essential saccharide shortage lead to depression in susceptible individuals
and does supplementation alleviate the problem? Perhaps. Depression is complex, and no simple cause-and-effect relationship
has been established. Studies on glyconutrients and depression
have yet to be conducted, but we do know that glucose levels in
the brains of those with chronic depression,[25, 26] as well as those
with anorexia or bulimia,[27, 28] obsessive-compulsive disorder,[29]
and schizophrenia,[30] are often lower than in those without these
disorders; in manic-depression, however, both high and low glucose levels have been cited.[31, 32] In addition, studies link low
blood glucose with impulsiveness, acting-out behavior, and histri-
onic and narcissistic traits in males.[33]

Some researchers theorize that in serious psychiatric disorders, inflammatory proteins in the brain called cytokines disrupt insulin-glucose metabolism.[34] The result may be too much glucose utilization initially, followed by too little. Too much may result in the overstimulation of the autonomic nervous system, which regulates involuntary body processes, including breathing and digestion. Too little may lead to problems with the limbic system, the deep-brain structures that impact emotion and behavior.

*Suggested Use:* Whether glucose or any other saccharides can mitigate symptoms in psychiatric diseases hasn't been established. If you believe you have low blood sugar, consult your doctor.

Encouraging animal research suggests that glyconutrients and glycolipids improve learning, memory, and intelligence; lower anxiety levels; and enhance sleep. As today's neurological and psychiatric drugs treat only symptoms and have problematic side effects, in the future, as we learn more, supplementation with glyconutrients may prove particularly worthwhile.

## Chapter 15

# Reversing Heart Disease

*Lowering blood pressure and "bad" cholesterol and raising "good" cholesterol with glyconutrients.*

In imperial Rome, Nero feasted on mice dipped in honey and sprinkled with nuts. No one knew from cholesterol, no one cared terribly much about calories. People ate what they wanted—a fact of life that held true through the 1960s, when anorexia nervosa first entered mainstream consciousness. Still, for most of us, good, wholesome food meant whole milk and butter cookies, red meat, and bacon and eggs—of which, no doubt, Nero would have approved. But nutrition practices changed in the 1970s, as the emphasis switched from red meat to fresh, organic fruits and vegetables. By the mid-1980s, high fat was deemed the architect of heart disease and high cholesterol, spawning a generation of low-fat and compensatory high-sugar snacks that have only made us fatter.

I tend to look at the latest food findings with skepticism—the latest "good" food will no doubt be transmogrified into "bad" food over time. And in any event, I don't think there's a black-

and-white rule—food that's good for one person can be bad for another. For the time being, this is what we know about cholesterol that can't be debated: Cholesterol is a waxy alcohol found only in animals. It's an important nutrient that generates essential adrenal and sex hormones that we need to sustain life. It comes from foods and is generated within the body.

We're so conditioned to worrying about high cholesterol that it's hard to imagine that it can be too low, but it can be. Levels under 150 are associated with increases in cancers, infection, liver damage, malnutrition, hyperthyroidism, and violent suicide.[1, 2] Too-high cholesterol, of course, can lead to heart disease by offloading into blood-vessel walls. This laying down of cholesterol, or plaque, marks the first chapter in the development of atherosclerosis, the condition that can eventually lead to scarring, narrowing, and even closure of the arteries. Atherosclerosis is responsible for most heart attacks and strokes in America and as such is the leading cause of death in both men and women. Plaque can begin forming in early childhood. Autopsies on children as young as two often reveal arteries streaked with cholesterol.

Cholesterol is carried from place to place within the bloodstream by transporter proteins called LDLs, short for low-density lipoproteins, with the nickname of "bad" cholesterol; and HDLs, or high-density lipoproteins, the so-called good cholesterol. HDLs, in fact, help rid the body of excess cholesterol. A high-LDL, low-HDL ratio is associated with atherosclerosis, heart attacks, and strokes.

High LDL levels contribute to the laying down of plaque, as does an insult or an injury to the cells lining the inside of the arteries caused by free-radical insult or disease. Smoking, inactivity, high blood pressure, obesity, stress, genetic factors, poor diet, diabetes, and other chronic diseases contribute to heart-disease progression. More recently, herpes viruses and various bacteria, including *Helicobacter pylori*, the agent that causes some kinds of peptic ulcers, have been implicated.

Another potential culprit that has received a lot of play in the science community and the media is *Chlamydia pneumoniae*, a mycoplasma—a pathogen with characteristics of both viruses and bacteria that responds to antibiotic therapy. Researchers in Finland, Japan, the United States, and elsewhere have found *C. pneumoniae* in the aorta and major arteries in the heart and have demonstrated that *C. pneumoniae* infection frequently precedes atherosclerosis.[3] In other words, the chronic infection causes chronic vascular inflammation that eventually leads to atherosclerosis—and not the other way around. *C. pneumoniae* isn't just a problem for middle-aged and older patients; researchers have detected the organism in the vascular walls in teenagers.

Whatever the cause of the vascular inflammation, the result is injury to the delicate endothelial cells that line the blood vessels in the heart. These damaged blood vessels allow LDL cholesterol to leak out into the blood vessel wall. The result is inflammation and oxidation, which attracts macrophages. The macrophages gorge themselves on this LDL cholesterol; they are then called foam cells (so-named because of their peculiar foamy appearance).[4] Often overwhelmed by their efforts, they may be incapable of disposing of the cholesterol safely. When they die, they release their foamy contents, which are caustic and rich in free radicals that attack surrounding tissue. The free radicals in turn attract more macrophages to the site, stoking the inflammatory cycle and leading to scarring and atherosclerotic blood vessel disease, and, down the road, to heart attack, stroke, or pulmonary embolism.[5]

In general, total cholesterol levels of greater than 200 are undesirable. Actuarial studies show the increased risk of heart attack in individuals as their levels of blood cholesterol rise. Up until recently, exercise, weight loss, antioxidants, and medications had been the best hope for bringing down high cholesterol. But now there might be something else to add to the mix: glyconutrients.

As we've seen in previous chapters, glyconutrients have immunomodulating effects, enabling the body to quash viruses and bacteria that may cause or contribute to heart disease as well as to mitigate the symptoms of autoimmune conditions, symptoms that can lead to blood-vessel damage and heart disease. Glyconutrients generate antioxidants that squelch free radicals and prevent the formation of foam cells, thereby averting the development of plaque and progression to serious disease. In particular, glyconutrients restore the activity of an enzyme called glutathione peroxidase, which is responsible for generating glutathione, one of the cells' most important antioxidants.[6, 7, 8] And glyconutrients also increase superoxide dismutase (SOD), a potent enzyme that neutralizes free radicals in humans and animals.[9]

## HIGH CHOLESTEROL: A PATIENT'S SUCCESS

Ari is a successful forty-one-year-old businessman who works in the food-processing industry. He has a degree in biochemistry and an MBA from an Ivy League university. He rises early and goes to bed late, has a hard-driving work ethic, and is a self-described Type A personality. He feels well, is vigorous, and plays tennis on Sunday mornings. Yet this highly motivated, self-disciplined man can't bring himself to stick to the low-cholesterol diet that his doctor put him on. Ari just can't give up the junk food and marbled meat. He has risk factors for a heart attack: Ari's moderately high cholesterol teeters around 210, and his father died of a massive heart attack at sixty-one. Instead of changing his diet, Ari tried glyconutrients, a combination of 500 milligrams of powdered aloe extracts taken twice a day and 1 gram of cordyceps mushroom capsules taken twice a day. He takes no other medication except a multivitamin. Six weeks after starting glyconutrients, his cholesterol dropped to the normal range at 176. Six months later, it was 181 and has stayed in that vicinity in the year since.

Of course, I'm not advocating that people with high cholesterol and other risk factors for health disease continue eating unhealthful foods. But in Ari's case cordyceps and aloe extracts may have helped bring down his cholesterol—despite his less-than-ideal eating habits. Studies on cordyceps, aloe, and other glyconutrients substantiate Ari's experience (see below for studies and intake recommendations). If you are taking cholesterol-lowering medication, you must always consult your doctor before trying glyconutrients. Your cholesterol and drug dosage will need close monitoring.

# Cholesterol

### CORDYCEPS

Cordyceps reduces the free-radical lipoperoxides that choles-terol and certain other fats produce. Lipoperoxides can be mea-sured by tracking a chemical called plasma malondialdehyde, or MDA, which tends to be high in older people. But in a con-trolled study in which seniors took 3 grams of the cordyceps ex-tract Cs-4 daily for three months, their MDA levels dropped to the low levels of people in their teens and early 20s.[10]

In a double-blind, placebo-controlled study done in 1990, Chi-nese researchers examined the effects of Cs-4 on 273 patients with genetic hyperlipidemia, which means they were genetically outfitted with too many fats in their blood, including cholesterol and triglycerides (the chief component of fatty tissue).[11] After two months the group taking 3 grams of Cs-4 daily experienced a 17 percent drop in total cholesterol and a 27 percent gain in HDL (the "good" cholesterol); both were significant over con-trols. Although the Cs-4 group saw a bigger drop in triglycerides than did the controls, it wasn't a statistically significant difference.

*Suggested Use:* If you're taking cholesterol-lowering medica-tions, always consult your doctor before adding any glyconutrient supplement. He or she may need to monitor your cholesterol and drug dosage more closely. Do not take cordyceps if you are on blood-thinning medications or have a bleeding disorder unless under a physician's care. I recommend 3 to 6 grams of cordyceps or Cs-4 extract, in divided doses, with your doctor's approval. Maintenance intake: 1 to 3 grams daily, in divided doses.

### OTHER GLYCONUTRIENTS

Aloe and psyllium lower cholesterol, too. In a five-year controlled study of 5,000 patients with angina—chest pain caused by insuffi-cient blood flow to the heart from coronary artery disease— those participants given *Aloe vera* and Isabgol husks, a psyllium fiber that contains polysaccharides, achieved a marked reduction in total serum cholesterol, serum triglycerides, and total lipids, as well as an increase in HDL.[12] The clinical picture improved as well: frequency of angina attacks went down, and patients needed less medication, including drugs called beta-blockers, commonly used to treat heart disease. Interestingly, the patients who most benefited were diabetics. Other studies have confirmed psyllium's ability to lower LDL and decrease cholesterol absorption in men with high cholesterol.[13]

The polysaccharide beta-glucans in oat bran also brings down cholesterol. (Slow-cooked confers more benefit than instant.) Rice bran brings down cholesterol levels as well—again, it's the beta-glucans that do it. In one study, scientists found that in patients with moderately high cholesterol, 84 grams a day of either oat bran or rice bran decreased LDL and total cholesterol significantly in 78 percent of participants within six weeks.[14] Other studies have shown similar cholesterol-lowering effects in one month with 30 grams of barley bran daily.[15] The beta-glucans in mushrooms lower cholesterol as well: in controlled studies shiitake mushrooms have been found to reduce cholesterol, phospholipids (the fats found in the cell membranes), and triglyceride levels, as compared with controls.[16]

*Suggested Use:* Always get your doctor's approval before adding glyconutrients to your diet. With your doctor's okay, try one of the following: 500 milligrams of *Aloe vera* once or twice daily; psyllium fiber (Metamucil is probably the best-known brand, but they all do the job): 10 grams, twice daily; rice, oat, or barley bran: follow manufacturer's recommendations and your doctor's advice. Read labels carefully. To enhance flavor, some manufacturers add sweetener to brans, which diabetics and those watching their weight should avoid. If you combine two glyconutrients, cut your intake in half; in you combine three, cut the amount by two-thirds. If you experience cramping, gas, or diarrhea, lower your intake. Also, add slow-cooked oatmeal and cooked shiitake mushrooms to your diet.

## POLYSACCHARIDE K

In animal trials, glyconutrients have been shown to reverse fatty streaks, the plaque that is the hallmark of atherosclerosis. Researchers set out to establish polysaccharide K's effects on rabbits with established heart disease in a study conducted in 2000 at the First Military Medical University in China.[17] Rabbits with diet-induced high cholesterol received either polysaccharide K or placebo. By the end of the trial, both groups had experienced a significant drop in cholesterol, but the levels in the polysaccharide K group were far lower. In addition, lipoperoxides—destructive free radicals generated from oxidizing activity in deposited cholesterol—were appreciably lower in the rabbits on polysaccharide K than in the control rabbits. (Lipoperoxide levels normally *increase* in patients and laboratory animals with atherosclerosis.[18])

Polysaccharide K reduced free-radical damage in the rabbits with atherosclerosis, in part by protecting the macrophages from injury and thereby raising the bar on their ability to wolf down pathogens. The researchers also discovered that the animals given polysaccharide K had experienced a regression of fatty streaks in the heart: as compared with the control group, plaque in the polysaccharide K rabbits diminished by 46 percent. The scientists concluded that polysaccharide K was a promising treatment for atherosclerosis, as it enhanced antioxidant capability, improved the antioxidant/free-radical ratio, and decreased cholesterol.

*Suggested Use:* Until we have the results of human trials, we won't know if the glyconutrient is effective in lowering cholesterol in humans. Polysaccharide K does confer benefits on the immune system, but always check with your doctor before trying any glyconutrients, particularly if you are on cholesterol-lowering drugs. If your doctor approves, take 1 to 6 grams daily, in divided doses. Start at 1 gram and build up gradually.

## Fibrin

Some patients with heart disease have too much fibrin in their blood. As a result, the blood clots too easily, potentially leading to heart attacks and strokes unless treated with blood thinners like heparin. Some glyconutrients, including pectins, also help control blood fibrin. In one controlled study, male patients with high cholesterol who received 15 grams a day of pectin for four weeks showed significant changes in the architecture of the blood fibrin, as compared with controls. The fibrin became weak and permeable, as compared with controls, and less likely to form a clot.[19] Similarly, reishi and cordyceps mushrooms contain the blood thinner adenosine, a nucleotide, which is a unit of our DNA and may help protect against the clots that are common in heart disease.[20]

*Suggested Use:* Caution: Do not use pectins, cordyceps, or reishi extracts if you have a bleeding disorder. Consult your doctor before trying glyconutrients to reduce fibrin levels, particularly if you are already on blood-thinning medications such as heparin, Coumadin, or Plavix; NSAIDS like ibuprofen or Motrin, Cox-2 inhibitors like Vioxx and Celebrex; and aspirin. You need to be monitored closely because thinning the blood too much can cause hemorrhaging. Pectins: 5 grams, two to three times a day; reishi extract: 3 to 6 grams a day, in divided doses; cordyceps or Cs-4 extract: 3 to 6 grams a day, in divided doses. If you use two glyconutrients, halve the dose for each; for three glyconutrients, cut the dose by two-thirds. If fibrin levels become normal, cut your dose in half.

## Blood Pressure

Reishi mushrooms are effective in lowering blood pressure in hypertensive patients—but not in those with normal blood pressure. In a Japanese study of 53 patients, group one had high blood pressure; group two had normal or mildly elevated blood pressure.[21] Every day for six months, both groups took 1.5 grams of reishi extract. By the end of the trial the hypertensive group had experienced a significant drop in blood pressure, whereas the group with normal or near-normal blood pressure did not.

Research also supports maitake's ability to lower blood pressure. When Japanese scientists administered powdered maitake to naturally hypertensive rats for a week, their blood pressure dropped 45 to 65 points. That reduction remained stable until the researchers discontinued the glyconutrients, whereupon the rats' blood pressure spiked to pretreatment levels. The researchers restarted the rats on maitake powder, and once again, the rats' blood pressure declined.[22]

*Suggested Use:* 1.0 to 1.5 grams of reishi extract daily. Consult your doctor before taking reishi to lower blood pressure, particularly if you are already taking medications to do so. If your pressure drops too low, dizziness, weakness, and fainting may result. Caution: Consult your doctor before adding reishi extracts if you have a bleeding disorder or if you are taking a blood-thinning medication, as the mushroom can further thin the blood. Until human studies are conducted we won't know if maitake lowers blood pressure in humans. Adding cooked maitake mushrooms or extracts may, however, boost the workings of your immune system. Follow manufacturer's instructions and your doctor's advice.

## Heart Failure

Heart failure can be temporary or chronic and occurs when the heart fails to maintain adequate blood circulation. Symptoms include swelling, shortness of breath, and bluish discoloration of the skin from poor oxygenation of the blood. High blood pressure, infections, hyperthyroidism, atherosclerosis (cholesterol deposits in the arteries), and arteriosclerosis (thickening and hardening in the arteries) are major causes. Chinese researchers at Fu-Jian Medical College divided sixty-four chronic heart failure patients ages fifty-four to sixty-nine into two groups.[23, 24] Control patients received conventional drugs, including digoxin, hydrochlorothiazide, isosorbide dinitrate, furosemide, or dopamine. The treatment group received standard medication plus 3 to 4 grams of Cs-4 daily for twenty-six months.

At the end of that period, the scientists noted that those on glyconutrients registered a 66 percent improvement in shortness of breath, as compared with a 25 percent improvement for those on only conventional treatment. In addition, heart ultrasounds revealed that Cs-4–treated patients had significantly greater improvements in their heart function than did those on just conventional treatments. Cs-4 patients also noted an improvement in their sense of well-being and ability to perform everyday activities; fatigue diminished and sexual drive increased.

*Suggested Use:* Patients in heart failure should always be under a doctor's care. A doctor must determine whether a patient can take glyconutrients because they can affect requirements of drugs; patients need to be closely monitored. Caution: In addition, cordyceps and Cs-4 extracts can cause bleeding problems in patients on blood thinners. Follow your doctor's advice.

Glyconutrients help tackle the problem of high cholesterol and coronary artery disease, as they can

- Reduce the absorption of cholesterol from the gut.
- Reduce LDL, the "bad" cholesterol.
- Increase HDL, the "good" cholesterol.
- Lower triglycerides.
- Decrease free radicals and foam cells.
- Increase powerful antioxidants, including glutathione and SOD.
- Trigger the healing process and the remodeling of tissues while reducing the formation of plaques.
- Lower blood pressure.
- Reduce angina pain.
- Relieve shortness of breath, fatigue, and other symptoms of heart failure.

## Chapter 16

# Prescription
# for the Future

*"We are not sensible of the most perfect health, as we are of the least sickness."* —Montaigne, French essayist, 1533–1592

When the Wright brothers flew the first motorized aircraft a distance less than the length of a modern Boeing 747 on a North Carolina field in 1903, most onlookers thought it was just a sideshow trick—very exciting to be sure, but of no lasting value. Others, however, began to imagine fleets of airships transporting people around the planet, soaring at high speed. From the ungainly aerial jerking of that fragile machine of wires, canvas, and wood they envisioned an immensely different, exhilarating future for the planet—our present.

Just as discoveries of natural laws have revolutionized other sciences, glyconutrients, I believe, are on the brink of revolutionizing the science of medicine. Although the scientific literature on essential saccharides is already vast, our overall understanding of glyconutrients is still developing. Nevertheless, we can now form good theories about why they work and formulate safe practices for using them. After all, more than a hundred years before vitamin C was identified in its molecular form, medical and practical people knew that something inside citrus fruits and raw potatoes prevented the deadly disease scurvy. They didn't know that a nutritional deficiency caused scurvy. They didn't even know about vitamin C, yet they knew enough to act. The fact is, we know more about essential saccharides today than our forefathers ever knew about vitamin C.

Knowledge emanates in part from asking the right questions. Western medicine continues to focus on illness rather than health, and thus asks: What causes diabetes? Why has the patient come down with tuberculosis or AIDS? How can we best manage angina attacks? The human body has been around for 120,000 years and has adapted to survive and thrive. Yet Western medicine looks at human beings from the disease paradigm: we ask questions about what causes disease rather than what causes health and why people stay healthy. Moreover, modern medicine doesn't treat the body's systems as a totality; instead it partitions the body into specialties and subspecialties. There is an apocryphal anecdote about an orthopedic surgeon, who, when questioned about the cardiovascular system, replied cavalierly that it was useful only as the pump to bring antibiotics to infected bone. Outside of that, heart and arteries were of no use to him.

This radical compartmentalizing of medicine is strictly a Western phenomenon, as is the concept of "rescue medicine"— attending to medical concerns after there's a problem, rather than preventing it from occurring in the first place. While I believe that most us of would be grateful to be rescued should an emergency occur, what we really want in terms of everyday living is to be as healthy as possible for as long as possible. Oriental, Ayurvedic (Indian), and traditional African doctors view the body in its entirety. There is elegance and simplicity in the communication and interreliance of all the cells in the body. Saccharides— the cells' communicators—help us work with our body as a whole.

Supplementing with glyconutrients can help in the body's

natural drive toward homeostasis and health. As we've seen in controlled studies in humans and animals, the saccharides in glyconutrients accelerate healing, improve immune functioning, help the body to fight cancer and pathogens, slow down aging, improve memory, lower anxiety, and quell autoimmune phenomena without toxic side effects. When health is improved or restored, mind and body shift over to what the Chinese call "the right side," embracing harmony, healing, and *gong*.

# Resources

## GLYCONUTRIENTS MENTIONED IN THE BOOK

**Active Hexose Correlated Compound (AHCC):** See AHCC Nutrients USA

**Aloe Vera:** See Academy Health, Carrington Labs, and Mannatech

**Arabinogalactans (Gum Sugars):** See Larex and Mannatech

**Bovine Tracheal Cartilage:** See EcoNugenics, Lescarden Inc., and Phoenix Biologics

**Chitin and Chitosan:** See Chitin and Chitosan section

**Glucosamine and Chondroitin:** See Nutramax Laboratories Inc.

**Inulin:** See Academy Health

**Lentinan:** See ITM (oral) and Injectable Lentinan (injectable)

**Mushrooms and Mushroom Extracts:** See EcoNugenics, The Farm, Fungi Perfecti, Gourmet Mushroom Products, ITM, JHN Natural Products, Maitake Products, MushroomScience, North American Reishi, PSP Extracts Inc., and Spanda

**Pectins:** See Academy Health and EcoNugenics

**Rice Bran:** See Lane Labs and NutraStar
**Yeast Beta-Glucans:** See ImmuDyne

## GLYCONUTRIENT SUPPLIERS

None of the three suppliers of bovine tracheal cartilage listed in the re-
source section use herds from Europe, where mad cow disease has been
documented. Lescarden uses cattle from Canada, the United States,
and New Zealand. EcoNugenics uses cattle from Australia. And Phoenix
Biologics' cattle comes from New Zealand and Australia. No cases of
people contracting mad cow disease from cattle have been documented
in the United States, Canada, New Zealand, or Australia. Cartilage contains no blood vessels or nerve cells, the areas in which mad cow disease
is most likely to be concentrated. However, the risk of contracting mad
cow disease from bovine tracheal cartilage, while unlikely, has not been
scientifically disproven.

ACADEMY HEALTH
80 High Street
Winchester
Hampshire
SO23 9AT
England
0044-(0)1256-773189
*www.academyhealth.com*
Inulin (from chicory), pectin (from grapefruit), *Aloe vera* products.
International shipping.

AHCC NUTRIENTS USA
22 East Lake Avenue
Watsonville, CA 95076
*http://ahcc-nutrients.com*
831-663-5327
Active Hexose Correlated Compound.

CARRINGTON LABS
2001 Walnut Hill Lane
Irving, TX 75038
800-444-ALOE
*www.aloevera.com*
*Aloe vera* products, including a skin-care line, several wound dressings

(including those for diabetic wounds and for patients receiving radiation or chemotherapy), and dietary supplements containing aloe. International shipping.

## ECONUGENICS
2208 Northpoint Parkway
Santa Rosa, CA 95407
800-308-5518
*www.econugenics.com*
Bovine cartilage, citrus pectin, mushroom-blend extracts. International shipping.

## THE FARM
c/o Mushroompeople
P.O. Box 220
Summertown, TN 38483-0220
800-692-6329; 931-964-2200
*www.mushroompeople.com*
Dried shiitake mushrooms, maitake and reishi extracts, mushroom kits and spawn (shiitake, maitake, oyster, reishi), instructional videos, books, and other supplies. International shipping.

## FUNGI PERFECTI
P.O. Box 7634
Olympia, WA 98507
800-780-9126 (U.S. and Canada); 360-426-9292
*www.fungiperfecti.com*
Dried mushrooms (reishi, maitake, shiitake, cordyceps) and freeze-dried capsules, including reishi, maitake, and cordyceps. Also tinctures (liquid form with alcohol), plus teas, mushroom-blend extracts, mushroom powders available in bulk, mushroom-growing kits, books, and mushroom seminars. International shipping.

## GOURMET MUSHROOM PRODUCTS
P.O. Box 515
Graton, CA 95444
800-789-9121; 707-829-7301
*www.gmushrooms.com*
Dried mushrooms (shiitake, reishi, and other gourmet mushrooms), fresh mushrooms (oyster, shiitake, among others), mushroom sauces, mushroom books, mushroom-growing kits. International shipping.

## IMMUDYNE
11200 Wilcrest Green Drive
Houston, TX 77042
888-246-6839;713-783-7034
*www.immudyne.com*
Beta-glucans (from yeast) in caplets, sunscreen, and moisturizer. International shipping.

## INJECTABLE LENTINAN
Injectable lentinan is a prescription drug and must be administered by a physician. When lentinan is administered by injection or intravenously, serious side effects have occurred, and they include anaphylaxis, a potentially fatal allergic reaction. For more information on obtaining injectable lentinan, have your physician contact either of these companies:

- Ajinomoto Ltd., Yokohama, Japan. Call 81-3-5250-8133 or visit the website (mostly in Japanese) at *www.ajinomoto.co.jp.*
- Eureka Bio-Chemicals, H/O Level 10, 114 Albert Road, South Melbourne 3205, Australia. Call 61-3-9525-0774 or visit *www.bio-chem.com.*

## ITM
2017 S.E. Hawthorne Blvd.
Portland, OR 97214
800-544-7504
*www.itmonline.org* (informational site only; call for orders)
Lentinan powder, reishi. International shipping.

## JHN NATURAL PRODUCTS
P.O. Box 50398
Eugene, OR 97405
1-888-330-4691
*www.jhsnp.com*
Polysaccharide K, polysaccharide P, reishi, cordyceps, mushroom-blend formula. International shipping.

## LANE LABS
P.O. Box 710
Saddle River, NJ 07458
800-510-2010
*www.lanelabs.com*
MGN-3: Pure rice bran and mushroom mix in capsule form. International shipping.

## LAREX
4815 White Bear Parkway
White Bear Lake, MN 55110
800-386-5300; 651-636-2628 (international orders)
*www.larex.com*
Arabinogalactans. International shipping.

## LESCARDEN INC.
Suite 212
420 Lexington Avenue
New York, NY 10170
888-581-2076
*www.catrix.com*
Bovine tracheal cartilage supplements and bovine tracheal cartilage wound dressing. International shipping.

## MAITAKE PRODUCTS
P.O. Box 1354
Paramus, NJ 07653
800-747-7418
*www.maitake.com*
Whole maitake caplets, maitake extracts (liquid and capsules), maitake D-fraction, mushroom-blend extracts, maitake tea. International shipping.

## MANNATECH
600 South Royal Lane, Suite 200
Coppell, TX 75019
*www.mannatech-inc.com* (check website for phone numbers and e-mail addresses of company associates in your area)
Ambrotose, which includes the eight essential saccharides from *Aloe vera*, larch arabinogalactans, and other gum sugars, in powder form or capsules, and AmbroDerm, a skin lotion. International shipping.

## MUSHROOMSCIENCE
P.O. Box 50398
Eugene, OR 97405
888-283-6583; 541-344-8753
*www.mushroomscience.com*
*Coriolus versicolor,* reishi, cordyceps, mushroom-blend extracts. International shipping.

## NORTH AMERICAN REISHI

Box 1780

Gibson BC V0N1V0

Canada

604-886-7799

*www.namex.com*

Reishi, shiitake, maitake, cordyceps, *Coriolus versicolor.* Whole mushrooms and mushroom powder, supplements. International shipping.

## NUTRAMAX LABORATORIES INC.

2208 Lakeside Boulevard

Edgewood, MD 21040

800-925-5187 (in U.S. and Canada)

*www.cosamin.com*

Glucosamine and chondroitin products for people and animals. International shipping.

## NUTRASTAR

1261 Hawk's Flight Court

Eldorado, CA 95762

877-723-1700

*www.nutrastar.com*

Four rice bran mixtures in bulk. Contains other nutrients. Check manufacturer's labels. International shipping.

## PHOENIX BIOLOGICS

2794 Loker Avenue West, Suite 104

Carlsbad, CA 92008

800-947-8482

*www.vitacarte.com*

Bovine tracheal cartilage. International shipping.

## PSP EXTRACTS INC.

138-5751 Cedarbridge Way

Richmond, BC V6X 2A8

Canada

604-241-9655

*www.psp.bc.ca*

Polysaccharide P, Cs-4, reishi extracts. International shipping.

SPANDA
823 North Street
Pittsfield, MA 01201
800-772-6320
*www.spanda.com*
Maitake mushroom caplets, maitake D-fraction, dried maitake mushrooms, teas, mushroom-blend extracts. International shipping.

## CHITIN AND CHITOSAN

Many companies make chitosan, including the Vitamin Shoppe, Keats Publishing, Only Natural Inc., Kal, Advanced Research, Ultimate Nutrition, Allergy Research Group, NutraSense, Natural Balance, and Source Naturals. Better health-food stores stock chitosan supplements. For more information, contact the Vitamin Shoppe at *www.vitaminshoppe.com* or 1-800-223-1216. Pure chitin is available only for commercial use, but you can make your own with the following recipes that are popular in Southern Cameroons, where I was raised.

**Kokee Corn**
    10 ears of fresh sweet corn (preferably yellow)
    4 ripe tomatoes
    4 tablespoons palm oil
    1 cup *njanga* (tiny shrimp with shells intact, available at Chinese and African groceries)
    4 bouillon cubes, crumbled
    1 cup thawed frozen, chopped spinach
    Plantain leaves (obtainable in Latino grocery stores) or aluminum foil for rolling (length: 18 inches for each rollup)
    ½ small, red-hot Jamaican pepper (optional)
Cut corn kernels from cobs. (Just run the knife lengthwise along the cob.) Blend with a fork lightly so that the pieces of corn are broken up and mushy, but not into a fine paste. Process tomatoes in a blender until they form a paste, and fold in corn. Remove seeds and stem from the Jamaican pepper and add half of it to the mixture if you want the kokee spicy. Add the palm oil, *njanga,* bouillon cubes, and spinach. Mix well. Lay the plantain leaves (they are fairly large) or 18-inch-long aluminum sheets flat on prep table. Scoop out 2 to 3 tablespoons of the mixture onto each sheet or leaf. Roll up cigar-style, and fold the ends in to hold in the mixture. Place bundles in a steamer with boiling water and cook, covered, over high heat for 1 hour. Check every 15 minutes to make

sure there's still water in the pot. Add more boiling water if necessary. Allow to cool. Unwrap aluminum foil before serving (the plantain leaves are edible). Serve as a meal (2 bundles per person) or side dish. Makes 10 to 12 bundles.

**N'dole Vegetable Sauce**
   1 medium onion, chopped
   3 ripe medium tomatoes
   4 garlic cloves
   2-inch slice of fresh ginger
   ½ small, red-hot Jamaican pepper (optional)
   ½ to 1 cup peanuts
   3 tablespoons vegetable oil
   3 bouillon cubes, crumbled
   Salt to taste
   3 boxes frozen chopped spinach or 4 bundles fresh spinach. (In Africa, we use leaves from a shrub called "bitter leaf")
   1 cup of *njanga* (tiny shrimp)
   1 pound cubed smoked turkey or ¼ pound diced cooked beef, or 1 pound cooked shelled shrimp

In a blender, combine the onion, tomatoes, garlic, and ginger and process to a paste. Add the Jamaican pepper to the mixture if you want the sauce spicy, first removing seeds and stem. Put mixture aside. Process peanuts in a blender separately into smooth paste. Heat oil in a large saucepan and add onion-tomato paste. Cook until most of water evaporates. Add the peanut paste to the mixture and cook over medium heat until peanuts release their oil. Add the bouillon cubes and salt to taste. Add spinach, *njanga,* and turkey, beef, or shrimp. Cook, stirring intermittently, for 5 minutes. Serve with rice, yams, or fried plantains. Serves 4-6 people.

## SUGGESTED READING

### BOOKS

Hall, S. *A Commotion in the Blood: Life, Death, and the Immune System.* New York: Henry Holt, 1997, 1998 (paperback).

Halpern, G. M. *Cordyceps: China's Healing Mushroom.* Garden City Park, NY: Avery Publishing Group, 1998.

Hobbs, C. *Medicinal Mushrooms: An Exploration of Tradition, Healing, and Culture.* Santa Cruz, CA: Botanica Press, 1995.

Johnson, H. *Osler's Web: Inside the Labyrinth of the Chronic Fatigue Syndrome Epidemic.* New York: Crown Publishers, 1996.

Jones, K. *Shiitake: The Healing Mushroom.* Rochester, VT: Inner Traditions, 1994.

Moore, N. *The Missing Link: The Facts About Glyconutrients.* Seattle, WA: Validation Press, 1997.

Regush, N. *The Virus Within: The Coming Epidemic.* New York: Dutton, 2000.

### REVIEW ARTICLES

Borchers, A. T., Stern, J. S., Hackman, R. M., et al. "Mushrooms, Tumors and Immunity." *Proceedings of the Society for Experimental Biology and Medicine* 221: 287, 1999.

Kidd, P. "The Use of Mushroom Glucans and Proteoglycans in Cancer Treatment." *Alternative Medicine Review* 5(1): 4–27, 2000.

Reynolds, T, and Dweck, A. C. "*Aloe vera* Leaf Gel: A Review Update." *Journal of Ethnopharmacology* 68(1-3): 3–37, 1999.

Zhu J. S., Halpern, G., and Jones, K. "The Scientific Rediscovery of an Ancient Chinese Herbal Medicine: *Cordyceps Sinensis.* Part I." *Journal of Alternative and Complementary Medicine* 4(3):289–303, 1998.

Zhu J. S., Halpern G., and Jones, K. "The Scientific Rediscovery of an Ancient Chinese Herbal Medicine: *Cordyceps Sinensis.* Part II." *Journal of Alternative and Complementary Medicine* 4(4):429–457, 1998.

### WEBSITES

*http://www.ncbi.nlm.nih.gov/PubMed:* Pub Med, a medical database. Abstracts are free.

*www.mushrooms.com:* Information, recipes, and links to other mushroom websites, including companies that sell mushrooms and extracts.

*www.silverplatter.com:* A comprehensive computer database that includes alternative medicine studies not found in standard medical databases. Membership fee required.

*www.SugarsThatHeal.org:* Noncommercial site with information on glyconutrients.

# Notes

## 1 COLEY'S SACCHARIDES

1. Hall S: *A Commotion in the Blood: Life, Death, and the Immune System.* New York: Henry Holt, 1997, 1998 (paperback), pp. 22–26, 38–42.
2. Narkia M: Coley's Toxins/Issel's Fever Therapy. URL: http://cancerguide.org/coley.html.
3. Narkia.
4. Hall.
5. Hall, p. 62.
6. Hall, pp. 118–122.
7. Bradova: URL: http://www.geocities.com:0080/~vera_b/alts/coley.html.
8. Hall, p. 107.
9. Bradova: URL: http://www.geocities.com:0080/~vera_b/alts/coley.html.
10. Hall, p. 104.
11. Hall, p. 102.

12. Hall, p. 104.
13. Macklis RM: Radithor and the era of mild radium therapy. *JAMA* 264(5):614–618, 1990.
14. Hall, pp. 76, 77.
15. Macklis.
16. Winslow R: The radium water worked fine until his jaw came off. *Wall Street Journal,* Aug 1, 1990, pp. A-1, A-5.
17. Winslow, p. A-5.
18. Winslow, p. A-5.
19. Macklis RM: The great radium scandal. *Scientific American,* Aug 1993, pp. 94–99.
20. Lackovic V; Borecky L; Sikl D; Masler L; Bauer S: Stimulation of interferon production by mannans. *Proc Soc Exp Biol Med* 134(3): 874–879, 1970.
21. Borecky L; Lackovic V; Blaskovic D; Masler L; Sikl D: An interferon-like substance induced by mannans. *Acta Virol* 11(3):264–266, 1967.
22. Hall, p. 116.
23. Chihara G: Recent progress in immunopharmacology and therapeutic effects of polysaccharides. *Dev Biol Stand* 77:191–197, 1992.
24. Sharon N; Lis H: Lectins as cell recognition molecules. *Science* 246 (Oct 13): 227–234, 1989.
25. Matsui H; Setogawa T; Naora H; Tanaka O: The effects of PSK, a biological response modifier, on congenital ocular abnormalities induced by X-ray irradiation. *Histol Histopathol* 10(1):47–54, 1995.
26. Kurishita A: Suppressive effects of two bioresponse modifiers, krestin and levamisole, on 5-azacytidine-induced digital defects in rats. *Teratog Carcinog Mutagen* 10(5):409–415, 1990.
27. Nishihira T; Akimoto M; Mori S: Anti-cancer effects of BRMs associated with nutrition in cancer patients. *Gan To Kagaku Ryoho* 15(4, Pt 2-3):1615–1620, 1988.

## 2  THE EIGHT ESSENTIAL SACCHARIDES

1. Weil A: *Spontaneous Healing.* New York: Ballantine Books, 1995, p. 184.
2. Ezekowitz RA; Stahl PD: The structure and function of vertebrate mannose lectin-like proteins. *J Cell Sci Suppl* 9:121–133, 1988.
3. Stahl PD; Ezekowitz RA: The mannose receptor is a pattern recognition receptor involved in host defense. *Curr Opin Immunol* 10(1):50–55, 1998.

4. Moore, N. *The Missing Link: The Facts About Glyconutrients.* Seattle, WA: Validation Press, 1997, pp. 56–57.

5. Bunyapraphatsara N; Yongchaiyudha S; Rungpitarasangsi V; et al.: Antidiabetic activity of *Aloe vera* L. juice. II. Clinical trial in diabetes mellitus patients in combination with glibenclamide. *Phytomedicine* 3(3):245–248, 1996.

6. Matthies H; Schroeder H; Smalla KH; Krug M: Enhancement of glutamate release by L-fucose changes effects of glutamate receptor antagonists on long-term potentiation in the rat hippocampus. *Learn Mem* 7(4):227–234, 2000.

7. Matthies H; Staak S; Krug M: Fucose and fucosyllactose enhance in-vitro hippocampal long-term potentiation. *Brain Res* 725(2): 276–280, 1996.

8. GlycoScience Nutrition Science Site. URL: http://www.usa.glycoscience.com.

9. Hoshino T; Hayashi T; Hayashi K; et al.: An antivirally active sulfated polysaccharide from *Sargassum horneri* (Turner) C. AGARDH. *Biol Pharm Bull* 21(7):730–734, 1998.

10. Baba T; Yoshida T; Yoshida T; Cohen S: Suppression of cell-mediated immune reactions by monosaccharides. *J Immunol* 122(3):838–841, 1979.

11. Beuth J; Ko HL; Schirrmacher V; et al.: Inhibition of liver tumor cell colonization in two animal tumor models by lectin blocking with d-galactose or arabinogalactan. *Clin Exp Metastasis* 6(2): 115–120, 1988.

12. Kodama T; Reddy VN; Giblin F; et al.: Scanning electron microscopy of X-ray-induced cataract in mice on normal and galactose diet. *Ophthalmic Res* 15(6):324–333, 1983.

13. Flögel M; Lauc G; Gornik I; Macek B: Fucosylation and galactosylation of IgG heavy chains differ between acute and remission phases of juvenile chronic arthritis. *Clin Chem Lab Med* 36(2):99–102, 1998.

14. Isenberg DA: Humoral immunity and glycosylation abnormalities in rheumatoid arthritis. *Clin Exp Rheumatol* 13(Suppl 12):S17–20, 1995.

15. Kötz K; Hänsler M; Sauer H; et al.: Immunoglobulin G galactosylation deficiency determined by isoelectric focusing and lectin affinoblotting in differential diagnosis of rheumatoid arthritis. *Electrophoresis* 17(3):533-534, 1996.

16. Tomana M; Schronhenloher RE; Reveille JD; et al.: Abnormal galactosylation of serum IgG in patients with systemic lupus

erythematosus and members of families with high frequency of autoimmune diseases. *Rheumatol Int* 12(5):191–194, 1992.

17. Crowe SF; Zhao WQ; Sedman GL; Ng KT: 2-Deoxygalactose interferes with an intermediate processing stage of memory. *Behav Neural Biol* 61(3):206–213, 1994.

18. Moore, pp. 102–104.

19. Bucht G; Adolfsson R; Lithner F; Winblad B: Changes in blood glucose and insulin secretion in patients with senile dementia of Alzheimer type. *Acta Med Scand* 213(5):387–392, 1983.

20. Itagaki T; Itoh Y; Sugai Y; et al.: Glucose metabolism and Alzheimer's dementia. *Nippon Ronen Igakkai Zasshi* 33(8):569–572, 1996.

21. Fujisawa Y; Sasaki K; Akiyama K: Increased insulin levels after OGTT load in peripheral blood and cerebrospinal fluid of patients with dementia of Alzheimer type. *Biol Psychiatry* 30(12):1219–1228, 1991.

22. Andreason PJ; Altemus M; Zametkin AJ; et al.: Regional cerebral glucose metabolism in bulimia nervosa. *Am J Psychiatry* 149(11): 1506–1513, 1993.

23. Martinot JL; Hardy P; Feline A; et al.: Left prefrontal glucose hypometabolism in the depressed state: a confirmation. *Am J Psychiatry* 147(10):313–317, 1990.

24. Delvenne V; Goldman S; De Maertelaer V; Lotstra F: Brain glucose metabolism in eating disorders assessed by positron emission tomography. *Int J Eat Disord* 25(1):29–37, 1999.

25. Moore, p. 172.

26. Moore, pp. 86, 87.

27. Deal CL; Moskowitz RW: Nutraceuticals as therapeutic agents in osteoarthritis. The role of glucosamine, chondroitin sulfate and collagen hydrolysate. *Rheum Dis Clin North Am* 25(2):379–395.

28. Setnikar I; Cereda R; Pacini MA; Revel L: Antireactive properties of glucosamine sulfate. *Arzneimittelforschung* 41:157–161, 1991.

29. Dunn AJ; Hogan EL: Brain gangliosides: Increased incorporation of (1-³H) glucosamine during training. *Pharmacol Biochem Behav* 3(4):605–612, 1975.

30. Murch SH; MacDonald TT; Walker-Smith JA; et al.: Disruption of sulphated glycosaminoglycans in intestinal inflammation. *Lancet* 341(8847):711–714, 1993.

31. Russell AL: Glycoaminoglycan (GAG) deficiency in protective barrier as an underlying, primary cause of ulcerative colitis, Crohn's disease, interstitial cystitis and possibly Reiter's syndrome. *Med Hypotheses* 52(4):297–301, 1999.

32. Morgan BL; Winick M: Effects of environmental stimulation on brain N-acetylneuraminic acid content and behavior. *J Nutr* 110(3): 425–432, 1980.

33. Woods JM; Bethell RC; Coates JA; et al.: 4-Guanidino-2,4dideoxy-2,3dehydro-N-acetylneuraminic acid is a highly effective inhibitor both of the sialidase (neuraminidase) and of growth of a wide range of influenza A and B viruses in vitro. *Antimicrob Agents Chemother* 37(7):1473–1479, 1993.

34. Ryan DM; Ticehurst J; Dempsey MH; Penn CR: Inhibition of influenza virus replication in mice by GG167 (4-guanidino-2,4-dideoxy-2,3-dehydro-N-acetylneuraminic acid) is consistent with extracellular activity of viral neuraminidase (sialidase). *Antimicrob Agents Chemother* 38(10):2270–2275, 1994.

35. Basset C; Durand V; Jamin C; et al.: Increased N-linked glycosylation leading to oversialylation of monomeric immunoglobulin A1 from patients with Sjögren's syndrome. *Scand J Immunol* 51(3): 300–306, 2000.

36. Sillanaukee P; Ponniö M; Seppä K: Sialic acid: New potential marker of alcohol abuse. *Alcohol Clin Exp Res* 23(6):1039–1043, 1999.

37. Moore, p. 140.

38. Dulkin LA: Absorption of carbohydrates in children with chronic enterocolitis. *Pediatriia* 9:33–36, 1991.

39. Lewis FW; Warren GH; Goff JS: Collagenous colitis with involvement of terminal ileum. *Dig Dis Sci* 36(8):1161–1163, 1991.

40. Fincher GB; Sawyer WH; Stone BA: Chemical and physical properties of an arabinogalactan-peptide from wheat endosperm. *Biochem J* 139(3):535–545, 1974.

41. Kelly GS: Larch arabinogalactan: Clinical relevance of a novel immune-enhancing polysaccharide. *Altern Med Rev* 4(2):96–103, 1999.

42. Hauer J; Anderer FA: Mechanism of stimulation of human natural killer cytotoxicity by arabinogalactan from *Larix occidentalis*. *Cancer Immunol Immunother* 36(4):237–244.

43. Hauer, Anderer, pp. 237–244.

44. Beuth J; Ko HL; Schirrmacher V; et al.: Inhibition of liver tumor cell colonization in two animal tumor models by lectin blocking with d-galactose or arabinogalactan. *Clin Exp Metastasis* 6(2):115–120, 1988.

45. Everson GT; Daggy BP; McKinley C; Story JA: Effects of psyllium hydrophilic mucilloid on LDL cholesterol and bile acid synthesis in hypercholesterolemic men. *J Lipid Res* 33(8):1183–1192, 1992.

46. Peterson JA; Patton S; Hamosh M: Glycoproteins of the human milk

fat globule in the protection of the breast-fed infant against infections. *Biol Neonate* 74(2):143–162, 1998.

47. McVeagh P; Miller JB: Human milk oligosaccharides: Only the breast. *J Paediatr Child Health* 33(4):281–286, 1997.

48. Jones K: Maitake: A potent medicinal food. *Altern Complement Ther,* Dec 1998, p. 420.

49. Laessoe T; Lincoff G: *Mushrooms.* New York: DK Publishing, 1998, p. 244.

50. Chiu JH; Ju CH; Wu LH; et al.: *Cordyceps sinensis* increases the expression of major histocompatibility complex class II antigens on human hepatoma cell line HA22T/VGH cells. *Am J Chin Med* 26(2):159–170, 1998.

51. Weil.

52. Zhu JS; Halpern GM; Jones K: The scientific rediscovery of an ancient Chinese herbal medicine: *Cordyceps sinensis.* Part I. *J Altern Complement Med* 4(3):289–303, 1998.

53. Borchers AT; Stern JS; Hackman RM; et al.: Mushrooms, tumors and immunity. *Proc Soc Exp Biol Med* 221:281–293, 1999.

54. Kurashige S; Akuzawa Y; Endo F: Effects of *Lentinus edodes, Grifola frondosa* and *Pleurotus ostreatus* administration on cancer outbreak, and activities of macrophages and lymphocytes in mice treated with a carcinogen, N-butyl-N-butanolnitrosamine. *Immunopharmacol Immunotoxicol* 19(2):175–183, 1997.

55. Wasser SP; Weis AL: Therapeutic effects of substances occurring in higher *Basidiomycetes* mushrooms: A modern perspective. *Crit Rev Immunol* 19(1):65–96, 1999.

56. Laessoe, p. 6.

57. Toth B; Erickson J: Cancer induction in mice by feeding of the uncooked cultivated mushroom of commerce *Agaricus bisporus. Cancer Res* 46(8):4007–4011, 1986.

58. Walton K; Walker R; Ionnides C: Effect of baking and freeze-drying on the direct and indirect mutagenicity of extracts from the edible mushroom *Agaricus bisporus. Food Chem Toxicol* 36(4):315–320, 1998.

59. Ghoneum M; Jewettt A: Production of tumor necrosis factor-alpha and interferon-gamma from human peripheral blood lymphocytes by MGN-3, a modified arabinoxylan from rice bran, and its synergy with interleukin-2 in vitro. *Cancer Detect Prev* 24(4):314–324, 2000.

60. Romano CF; Lipton A; Harvey HA; et al.: A phase II study of Catrix-S in solid tumors. *J Biol Response Mod* 4(6):585–589, 1985.

61. Puccio C; Mittelman A; Chun H; Baskind P; Ahmed T: Treatment of

metastatic renal cell carcinoma with Catrix. *Proc Annu Meet Am Soc Clin Oncol* 13:A769, 1994.

62. Shibata Y; Foster LA; Bradfield JF; Myrvik QN: Oral administration of chitin down-regulates serum IgE levels and lung eosinophilia in the allergic mouse. *J Immunol* 164(3):1314–1321, 2000.

63. Jong SC; Birmingham JM: Medicinal benefits of the mushroom *Ganoderma. Adv Appl Microbiol* 37:118, 1992.

64. van der Hem LG, van der Vliet JA; Bocken CF; et al.: Ling zhi-8: Studies of a new immunomodulating agent. *Transplantation* 60(5): 438–443, 1995.

65. Nanba H; Kubo K: Effect of maitake D-fraction on cancer prevention. *Ann N Y Acad Sci* 833:204–207, 1997.

66. Nanba H: Activity of maitake D-fraction to inhibit carcinogenesis and metastasis. *Ann N Y Acad Sci* 768:243–245, 1995.

## 3  NUTRIONAL SUPPLEMENTS

1. Fulder S: *The Book of Ginseng and Other Chinese Herbs for Vitality.* Rochester, VT: Healing Arts Press, 1993, pp. 63–64.

2. Veith I [trans]: *Huang Ti Nei Ching Su Wen: The Yellow Emperor's Classic of Internal Medicine.* Baltimore, MD: Williams & Wilkins, 1949.

3. Kurishita A: Suppressive effects of two bioresponse modifiers, krestin and levamisole, on 5-azacytidine-induced digital defects in rats. *Teratog Carcinog Mutagen* 10(5):409–415, 1990.

4. Matsui H; Setogawa T; Naora H; Tanaka O: The effects of PSK, a biological response modifier, on congenital ocular abnormalities induced by X-ray irradiation. *Histol Histopathol* 10(1):47–54, 1995.

## 4  INTRODUCTION TO THE IMMUNE SYSTEM

1. Ishihara Y; Fujii T; Iijima H; et al.: The role of neutrophils as cytotoxic cells in lung metastasis: Suppression of tumor cell metastasis by a biological response modifier (PSK). *In Vivo* 12(2):175–182, 1998.

2. Nathan CF: Secretory products of macrophages. *J Clin Invest* 79(2):319–326, 1987.

3. Lieu CW; Lee SS; Wang SY: The effect of *Ganoderma lucidum* on induction of differentiation in leukemic U937 cells. *Anticancer Res* 12(4):1211–1215, 1992.

4. Nanba H: Antitumor activity of orally administered "D-fraction" from maitake mushroom *(Grifola frondosa). J Naturopathic Med* 4(1):10–15, 1993.

5. Luettig B; Steinmüller G; Gifford GE; et al.: Macrophage activation by polysaccharide arabinogalactan isolated from plant cell cultures of *Echinacea purpura*. *J Natl Cancer Inst* 81(9):669–675, 1989.

6. Kim HS; Kacew S; Lee BM: In vitro chemopreventive effects of plant polysaccharides (*Aloe barbadensis miller, Lentinus edodes, Ganoderma lucidum* and *Coriolus versicolor*). *Carcinogenesis* 20(8):1637–1640, 1999.

7. Pang ZJ; Chen Y; Zhou M; Wan J: Effect of polysaccharide krestin on glutathione peroxidase gene expression in mouse peritoneal macrophages. *Br J Biomed Sci* 57(2):130–136, 2000.

8. Sabeh F; Wright T; Norton SJ: Purification and characterization of a glutathione peroxidase from the *Aloe vera* plant. *Enzyme Protein* 47(2):92–98, 1993.

9. Hassan IS; Bannister BA; Akbar A; et al.: A study of the immunology of the chronic fatigue syndrome: Correlation of immunologic parameters to health dysfunction. *Clin Immunol Immunopathol* 87(1): 60–67, 1998.

10. Vojdani A; Ghoneum M; Choppa PC; et al.: Elevated apoptotic cell population in patients with chronic fatigue syndrome: The pivotal role of protein kinase RNA. *J Intern Med* 242(6):465–478, 1997.

11. Liu C; Lu S; Ji MR: Effects of *Cordyceps sinensis* (CS) on in vitro natural killer cells. *Chung Kuo Chung Hsi I Chieh Ho Tsa Chih* 12(5): 267–269, 259, 1992.

12. Xu R; Peng X; Chen GZ; Chen GL: Effects of *Cordyceps sinensis* on natural killer activity and colony formation of $B_{16}$ melanoma. *Chinese Med J* 105(2):97–101, 1992.

13. Adachi K; Nanba H; Kuroda H; Kuroda H: Potentiation of host-mediated antitumor activity in mice by β-glucan obtained from *Grifola frondosa* (Maitake). *Chem Pharm Bull* 35(1):262–270, 1987.

14. Womble D; Helderman JH: The impact of acemannan on the generation and function of cytotoxic T-lymphocytes. *Immunopharmacol Immunotoxicol* 14(1-2):63–77, 1992.

15. Womble D; Helderman JH: Enhancement of allo-responsiveness of human lymphocytes by acemannan (Carrisyn). *Int J Immunopharmacol* 10(8):967–974, 1988.

16. Adachi et al., Host-mediated antitumor activity, pp. 262–270.

17. Adachi Y; Okazaki M; Ohno N; et al.: Enhancement of cytokine production by macrophages stimulated with (1→3)-β-D-glucan, grifolan (GRN), isolated from *Grifola frondosa*. *Biol Pharm Bull* 17(12): 1554–1560, 1994.

18. Adachi et al., Enhancement of cytokine production, pp. 1554–1560.
19. Chihara G; Hamuro J; Maeda YY; et al.: Antitumor and metastasis-inhibitory activities of lentinan as an immunomodulator: An overview. *Cancer Detect Prev Suppl* 1:423–443, 1987.

## 5 PREVENTING THE COMMON COLD AND OTHER VIRUSES

1. Tomassini JE; Maxson TR; Colonno RJ: Biochemical characterization of a glycoprotein required for rhinovirus attachment. *J Biol Chem* 264(3):1656–1662, 1989.
2. Saavedra J; Tschernia A; Moore N; et al.: Gastrointestinal function in infants consuming a weaning food supplemented with oligofructose, a prebiotic. *J Pediatr Gastroenterol Nutr* 29(4):95A, 1999.
3. Saavedra J; Tschernia A; Moore N; et al.: Effects of long-term consumption of a weaning food supplemented with oligofructose, a prebiotic, on general infant health status. *J Pediatr Gastroenterol Nutr* 29(4):58A, 1999.
4. Tsuru S: Depression of early protection against influenza virus infection by cyclophosphamide and its restoration by protein-bound polysaccharide. *Kitasato Arch Exp Med* 65(2-3):97–110, 1992.
5. Suzuki F; Suzuki C; Shimomura E; et al.: Antiviral and interferon-inducing activities of a new peptidomannan, KS-2, extracted from culture mycelia of *Lentinus edodes*. *J Antibiot* (Tokyo) 32(12): 1336–1345, 1979.
6. Chinnah AD; Baig MA; Tizard IR; Kemp MC: Antigen dependent adjuvant of a polydispersed beta (1,4)–linked acetylated mannan (acemannan). *Vaccine* 10(8):551–557, 1992.
7. Guangwen Y; Jianbin Y; Dongqin L; et al.: Immunomodulatory and therapeutic effect of lentinan in treating Condyloma acuminatum. *Chin J Integrated Traditional West Med* 5(3):190–192, 1999.
8. Williams RK; Straus SE: Specificity and affinity of binding of herpes simplex virus type 2 glycoprotein B to glycosaminoglycans. *J Virol* 71(2):1375–1380, 1997.
9. Marchetti M; Pisani S; Pietropaolo V; et al.: Antiviral effect of a polysaccharide from Sclerotium glucanicum towards herpes simplex virus type 1 infection. *Planta Med* 62(4):303–307, 1996.
10. Monma Y; Kawana T; Shimizu F: In vitro inactivation of herpes simplex virus by a biological response modifier, PSK. *Antiviral Res* 35(3):131–138, 1997.

11. Kim YS; Eo SK; Oh KW; et al.: Antiherpetic activities of acidic protein-bound polysaccharide isolated from *Ganoderma lucidum* alone and in combinations with interferons. *J Ethnopharmacol* 72:451–458, 2000.

12. Ebihara K; Minamishima Y: Protective effect of biological response modifiers on murine cytomegalovirus infection. *J Virol* 51(1): 117–122, 1984.

## 6 TREATING BACTERIAL, FUNGAL, AND PARASITIC INFECTIONS

1. Zopf D; Roth S: Oligosaccharide anti-infective agents. *Lancet* 347: 1017–1021, 1996.

2. Sharon N; Lis H: Carbohydrates in cell recognition. *Scientific American*, Jan 1993, p. 85.

3. Sharon, Lis, p. 85.

4. Sharon, Lis, p. 86.

5. Schaeffer AJ; Amundsen SK; Jones JM: Effect of carbohydrates on adherence of Escherichia coli to human urinary epithelial cells. *Infect Immun* 30(2):531–537, 1980.

6. Hibberd ML; Sumiya M; Summerfield JA; et al.: Association of variants of the gene for mannose-binding lectin with susceptibility to meningococcal disease. Meningococcal Research Group. *Lancet* 353(9158):1049–1053, 1999.

7. Uetsuka A; Satoh S; Ohno Y: Protective effect of PSK, a protein-bound polysaccharide preparation against candidiasis in tumor-bearing mice. *Adv Exp Med Biol* 121B:21–31, 1979.

8. Ghannoum MA; Abu-Elteen K; Ibrahim A; Stretton R: Protection against *Candida albicans* gastrointestinal colonization and dissemination by saccharides in experimental animals. *Microbios* 67(271): 95–105, 1991.

9. Stuart RW; Lefkowitz DL; Lincoln JA; et al.: Upregulation of phagocytosis and candidicidal activity of macrophages exposed to the immunostimulant acemannan. *Int J Immunopharmacol* 19(2):75–82, 1997.

10. Goldman R; Jaffe CL: Administration of beta-glucan following *Leishmania major* infection suppresses disease progression in mice. *Parasite Immunol* 13(2):137–145, 1991.

11. Luettig B; Steinmuller G; Gifford GE; et al.: Macrophage activation by the polysaccharide arabinogalactan isolated from plant cell cultures of *Echinacea purpura. J Natl Cancer Inst* 81(9):669–675, 1989.

12. Jones K: Maitake: A potent medicinal food. *Altern Complement Ther,* Dec 1998, p. 426.

13. Boroskova Z; Reiterova K; Dubinsky P; et al.: Inhibition of lymphoproliferative response and its restoration with a glucan immunomodulator in mice with experimental larval toxocarosis. *Folia Microbiol (Praha)* 43(5):475–476, 1998.

## 7 ALLEVIATING ALLERGIES, ASTHMA, AND OTHER PULMONARY DISEASES

1. Sharon N; Lis H: Lectins as cell recognition molecules. *Science* 246:227–234, 1989.

2. Shirakawa T; Enomoto T; Shimazu S; Hopkin JM: The inverse association between tuberculin responses and atopic disorder. *Science* 275(5296):77–79, 1997.

3. Shibata Y; Foster LA; Bradfield JF; Myrvik QN: Oral administration of chitin down-regulates serum IgE levels and lung eosinophilia in the allergic mouse. *J Immunol* 164(3):1314–1321, 2000.

4. Nogami M; Tsuji Y; Kubo M; et al.: Studies on *Ganoderma lucidum.* VI. Anti-allergic effect. *Yakugaku Zasshi* 106(7):594–599, 1986.

5. Jong SC; Birmingham JM: Medicinal benefits of the mushroom *Ganoderma. Adv Appl Microbiol* 37:118–119, 1992.

6. Kohda H; Tokumoto W; Sakamoto K; et al.: The biologically active constitutents of *Ganoderma lucidum* (fr.) karst. histamine release-inhibitory triterpenes. *Chem Pharm Bull* 33(4):1367–1374, 1985.

7. Tasaka K; Akagi M; Miyoshi M; et al.: Anti-allergic constituents in the culture medium of *Ganoderma lucidum.* (1) inhibitory effect of oleic acid on histamine release. *Agents and Actions,* Apr 23(304): 153–156, 1988.

8. Zhu JS; Halpern GM; Jones K: The scientific rediscovery of an ancient Chinese herbal medicine: *Cordyceps sinensis.* Part I. *J Altern Complement Med* 4(3):295–296, 1998.

9. Tekin D; Sin BA; Mungan D; Mirsirligil Z; Yavuzer S: The antioxidative defense in asthma. *J Asthma* 37(1):59–63, 2000.

10. Zhu, Halpern, Jones, Part I, p. 294.

11. Zhu JS; Halpern G; Jones K: The scientific rediscovery of a precious ancient Chinese herbal medicine: *Cordyceps sinensis.* Part II. *J Altern Complement Med* 4(4):430, 1998.

12. Zhu, Halpern, Jones, Part II, p. 430.

13. Jong, Birmingham, p. 118.

14. Shida T; Yagi A; Nishimura H; Nishioka I: Effect of aloe extract on peripheral phagocytosis in adult bronchial asthma. *Planta Medica* June(3):273–275, 1985.

15. Hobbs C: *Medicinal Mushrooms: An Exploration of Tradition, Healing & Culture.* Williams, OR: Botanica Press, 1995, p. 38.

## 8  HEALING SKIN DISORDERS, BURNS, AND WOUNDS

1. Updike J: *Self-Consciousness: Memoirs.* New York: Alfred Knopf, 1989, p. 48.

2. Updike, p. 45.

3. Kaufman T; Kalderon N; Ullmann Y; Berger J: *Aloe vera* gel hindered wound healing of experimental second-degree burns: A quantitative controlled study. *J Burn Care Rehabil* 9(2):156–159, 1988.

4. Schmidt JM; Greenspoon JS: *Aloe vera* dermal wound gel is associated with a delay in wound healing. *Obstet Gynecol* 78(1):115–117, 1991.

5. Syed TA; Ahmad SA; Holt AH; et al.: Management of psoriasis with *Aloe vera* extract in a hydrophilic cream: A placebo-controlled, double-blind study. *Trop Med Int Health* 1(4):505–509, 1996.

6. Beers MH; Berkow R (eds): *The Merck Manual: Diagnosis and Therapy.* 17th Ed (Centennial Edition). Whitehouse Station, NJ: Merck, 1999, p. 789.

7. Vardy DA; Cohen AD; Tchetov T; et al.: A double-blind placebo-controlled trial of an *Aloe vera (A. Barbadensis)* emulsion in the treatment of seborrheic dermatitis. *J Dermatol Treat* 10:7–11, 1999.

8. Visuthikosol V; Chowchuen B; Sukwanarat Y; et al.: Effect of *Aloe vera* gel to healing of burn wound: A clinical and histologic study. *J Med Assoc Thai* 78(8):403–409, 1995.

9. Tanzi E; Perez M: The effects of Catrix 10 ointment on laser resurfaced facial skin. American Society for Dermatologic Surgery Annual Meeting, Nov 2–5, 2000.

10. Tizard IR; Busbee D; Maxwell B; Kemp MC: Effects of acemannan, a complex carbohydrate, on wound healing in young and aged rats. *Wounds* 6:201–209, 1994.

11. Davis RH; Leitner MG; Russo JM; Byrne ME: Wound healing. Oral and topical activity of *Aloe vera. J Am Podiatr Med Assoc* 79(11): 559–562, 1989.

12. Ramamoorthy L; Kemp MC; Tizard IR: Acemannan, a beta-(1,4)-acetylated mannan, induces nitric oxide production in macrophage cell line RAW 264.7. *Mol Pharmacol* 50(4):878–884, 1996.

13. Chithra P; Sajithlal GB; Chandrakasan G: Influence of *Aloe vera* on collagen turnover in healing of dermal wounds in rats. *Indian J Exp Biol* 36(9):896–901, 1998.

14. Rodriguez-Bigas M; Cruz NI; Suarez A: Comparative evaluation of *Aloe vera* in the management of burn wounds in guinea pigs. *Plast Reconstr Surg* 81(3):386–389, 1988.

15. Heggers JP; Kucukcelebi A; Listengarten D; et al.: Beneficial effect of aloe on wound healing in an excisional wound model. *J Altern Complement Med* 2(2):271–277, 1996.

16. Heggers, Kucukcelebi, Listengarten, pp. 271–277.

17. Davis RH; Donato JJ; Hartman GM; Haas RC: Anti-inflammatory and wound healing activity of a growth substance in *Aloe vera. J Am Podiatr Med Assoc* 84(2):77–81, 1994.

18. Davis RH; DiDonato JJ; Johnson RW; Stewart CB: Aloe vera, hydrocortisone, and sterol influence on wound tensile strength and anti-inflammation. *J Am Podiatr Med Assoc* 84(12):614–621, 1994.

19. Fulton JE: The stimulation of postdermabrasion wound healing with stabilized *Aloe vera* gel-polyethylene oxide dressing. *J Dermatolo Surg Oncol,* May 16(5):460–467, 1990.

## 9  ADDRESSING CHRONIC FATIGUE SYNDROME, FIBROMYALGIA, AND GULF WAR SYNDROME

1. Jones K: Reishi mushroom: Ancient medicine in modern times. *Altern Complement Ther,* Aug 1998, p. 258.

2. Jones, p. 258.

3. Whiteside TL; Fridberg D: Natural killer cells and natural killer cell activity in chronic fatigue syndrome. *Am J Med* 105(3A):27S–34S, 1998.

4. Johnson H: *Osler's Web: Inside the Labyrinth of the Chronic Fatigue Syndrome Epidemic.* New York: Crown Publishers, 1996, p. 10.

5. Johnson, p. 10.

6. Urnovitz HB; Tuite JJ; Higashida JM; Murphy WH: RNAs in the sera of Persian Gulf War veterans have segments homologous to chromosome 22q11.2. *Clin Diagn Lab Immunol* 6(3):330–335, 1999.

7. Zhang Q; Zhou XD; Denny T; et al.: Changes in immune parameters seen in Gulf War veterans but not in civilians with chronic fatigue syndrome. *Clin Diagn Lab Immunol* 6(1):6–13, 1999.

8. Lekander M; Fredrikson M; Wik G: Neuroimmune relations in

patients with fibromyalgia: A positron emission tomography study. *Neurosci Lett* 282(3):193–196, 2000.

9. Demitrack MA; Dale JK; Straus SE; et al.: Evidence for impaired activation of the hypothalamic-pituitary-adrenal axis in patients with chronic fatigue syndrome. *J Clin Endocrinol Metab* 73:1224–1234, 1991.

10. Johnson, p. 131.

11. Shilts R: *And the Band Played On: Politics, People and the AIDS Epidemic*. New York: St. Martin's Press, 2000 (paperback).

12. Hassan IS; Bannister BA; Akbar A; et al.: A study of the immunology of the chronic fatigue syndrome: Correlation of immunologic parameters to health dysfunction. *Clin Immunol Immunopathol* 87(1): 60–67, 1998.

13. Vojdani A; Ghoneum M; Choppa PC; et al.: Elevated apoptotic cell population in patients with chronic fatigue syndrome: The pivotal role of protein kinase RNA. *J Intern Med* 242(6):465–478, 1997.

14. Hauer J; Anderer FA: Mechanism of stimulation of human natural killer cytotoxicity by arabinogalactan from *Larix occidentalis*. *Cancer Immunol Immunother* 36(4): 237–244, 1993.

15. Liu C; Lu S; Ji MR: Effects of *Cordyceps sinensis* (CS) on in vitro natural killer cells. *Chung Kuo Chung Hsi I Chieh Ho Tsa Chih* 12(5): 267–269, 259, 1992.

16. Xu R; Peng X; Chen GZ; Chen GL: Effects of *Cordyceps sinensis* on natural killer activity and colony formation of $B_{16}$ melanoma. *Chin Med J* 104(1):97–101, 1992.

17. Ghoneum M; Jewettt A: Production of tumor necrosis factor-alpha and interferon-gamma from human peripheral blood lymphocytes by MGN-3, a modified arabinoxylan from rice bran, and its synergy with interleukin-2 in vitro. *Cancer Detect Prev* 24(4):314–324, 2000.

18. Adachi K; Nanba H; Juroda H: Potentiation of host-mediated antitumor activity in mice by β-glucan obtained from *Grifola frondosa* (Maitake). *Chem Pharm Bull* 35(1):262–270, 1987.

19. Aoki T; Usuda Y; Miyakoshi H; Tamura K: Low natural killer syndrome: Clinical and immunologic features. *Nat Immun Cell Growth Regul* 6:116–128, 1987.

20. Uchida A: Chronic fatigue immune dysfunction syndrome. *Nippon Rinsho* 50(11):2625–2629, 1992.

21. Tsuru S: Depression of early protection against influenza virus infection by cyclophosphamide and its restoration by protein-bound polysaccharide. *Kitasato Arch Exp Med* 65(2-3):97–110, 1992.

22. Ando T; Motokawa I; Sakurai K; et al.: Effects of PSK on resistance

to bacterial infection in splenectomized mice. *Oncology* 45(3): 224–229, 1988.

23. Sabolovic D; Galoppin L: Effect of a protein bound polysaccharide (PSK) on tumor development and infections in splenectomized rats and mice. *Int J Immunopharmacol* 8(1):41–46, 1986.

24. Uetsuka A; Satoh S; Ohno Y: Protective effect of PSK, a protein-bound polysaccharide preparation against candidiasis in tumor-bearing mice. *Adv Exp Med Biol* 121B:21–31, 1979.

25. Ghannoum MA; Abu-Elteen K; Ibrahim A; Stretton R: Protection against *Candida albicans* gastrointestinal colonization and dissemination by saccharides in experimental animals. *Microbios* 67(271): 95–105, 1991.

26. Richards RS; Roberts TK; Dunstan RH; et al.: Free radicals in chronic fatigue syndrome: Cause or effect? *Redox Rep* 5(2–3): 146–147, 2000.

27. Zhu JS; Halpern GM; Jones K: The scientific rediscovery of an ancient Chinese herbal medicine: *Cordyceps sinensis*. Part I. *J Altern Complement Med* 4(3):295, 1998.

28. Pang ZJ; Chen Y; Zhou M; Wan J: Effect of polysaccharide krestin on glutathione peroxidase gene expression in mouse peritoneal macrophages. *Br J Biomed Sci* 57(2):130–136, 2000.

29. Sabeh F; Wright T; Norton SJ: Purification and characterization of a glutathione peroxidase from the *Aloe vera* plant. *Enzyme Protein* 47(2):92–98, 1993.

30. Kim HS; Kacew S; Lee BM: In vitro chemopreventive effects of plant polysaccharides (*Aloe barbadensis miller, Lentinus Edodes, Ganoderma lucidum* and *Coriolus versicolor*). *Carcinogenesis* 20(8):1637–1640, 1999.

31. Hayashi K; Hayashi T; Kojima I: A natural sulfated polysaccharide, calcium spirulan, isolated from Spirulina platensis: In vitro and ex vivo evaluation of anti-herpes simplex virus and anti-human immunodeficiency virus activities. *AIDS Res Hum Retroviruses* 12(15): 1463–1471, 1996.

32. Kelly GS: Larch arabinogalactan: Clinical relevance of a novel immune-enhancing polysaccharide. *Altern Med Rev* 4(2):96–103, 1999.

33. Ebihara K; Minamishima Y: Protective effect of biological response modifiers on murine cytomegalovirus infection. *J Virol* 51(1): 117–122, 1984.

34. Ebihara, Minamishima, pp. 117–122.

35. Williams RK; Straus SE: Specificity and affinity of binding of herpes

simplex virus type 2 glycoprotein to glycosaminoglycans. *J Virol* 71(2):1375–1380, 1997.

36. Marchetti M; Pisani S; Pietropaolo V; et al.: Antiviral effect of a polysaccharide from *Sclerotium glucanicum* towards herpes simplex virus type 1 infection. *Planta Med* 62(4):303–307, 1996.

37. Monma Y; Kawana T; Shimizu F: In vitro inactivation of herpes simplex virus by a biological response modifier, PSK. *Antiviral Res* 35(3):131–138, 1997.

38. Cuende JI; Civeira P; Diez N; Prieto J: High prevalence without reactivation of herpes virus 6 in subjects with chronic fatigue syndrome. *An Med Interna* 14(9):441–444, 1997.

39. Regush N: *The Virus Within: The Coming Epidemic.* New York: Dutton, 2000, p. 225.

40. Ablashi DV; Eastman HB; Owen CB; et al.: Frequent HHV-6 reactivation in multiple sclerosis (MS) and chronic fatigue syndrome (CFS) patients. *J Clin Virol* 16(3):179–191, 2000.

41. Stratton CW; Mitchell WM; Sriram S: Does *Chlamydia pneumoniae* play a role in the pathogenesis of multiple sclerosis? *J Med Microbiol* 49(1):1–3, 2000.

42. Nasralla M; Haier J; Nicolson GL: Multiple mycoplasmal infections detected in blood of patients with chronic fatigue syndrome and/or fibromyalgia syndrome. *Eur J Clin Microbiol Infect Dis* 18(12): 859–865, 1999.

43. Nicolson GL; Rosenberg-Nicolson NL: Doxycycline treatment and Desert Storm. *JAMA* 273(8):618–619, 1995.

44. Klapow LA: Roundworm-like specimens in the sputum of Chronic Fatigue Syndrome patients and controls in open and blind analysis [abstract]. Presented at the bi-annual research conference of the American Association for Chronic Fatigue Syndrome (AACFS), Oct 10–11, 1998, Cambridge, Mass. URL: http://www.cifds-me.org/aacfs/poster5.html#klapow.

45. Goldman R; Jaffe CL: Administration of beta-glucan following *Leishmania major* infection suppresses disease progression in mice. *Parasite Immunol* 13(2):137–145, 1991.

46. Boroskova Z; Reiterova K; Dubinsky P; et al.: Inhibition of lymphoproliferative response and its restoration with a glucan immunomodulator in mice with experimental larval toxocarosis. *Folia Microbiol (Praha)* 43(5):475–476, 1998.

47. Borish L; Schmaling K; DiClementi JD; et al.: Chronic fatigue syndrome: Identification of distinct subgroups on the basis of allergy

and psychologic variables. *J Allergy Clin Immunol* 102(2):222–230, 1998.

48. Rook GA; Zumla A: Gulf War syndrome: Is it due to a systemic shift in cytokine balance towards a Th2 profile? *Lancet* 349(9068): 1831–1833, 1997.

49. Hader N; Rimon D; Kinarty A; Lahat N: Altered interleukin-2 secretion in patients with primary fibromyalgia syndrome. *Arthritis Rheum* 34(7):866–872, 1991.

50. Barker E; Fujimura SF; Fadem MB; et al.: Immunological abnormalities associated with chronic fatigue syndrome. *Clin Infect Dis* 18 (suppl 1):S136–141, 1994.

51. Matsumoto Y; Ninomiya S: Allergy among Japanese patients with a chronic fatigue syndrome. *Arerugi* 41(12):1722–1725, 1992.

52. Rook, Zumla, pp. 1831–1833.

53. Sathyamoorthy N; Decker JM; Sherblom AP; Muchmore A: Evidence that specific high mannose structures directly regulate multiple cellular activities. *Mol Cell Biochem* 102(2):139–147, 1991.

54. Womble D; Helderman JH: The impact of acemannan on the generation and function of cytotoxic T-lymphocytes. *Immunopharmacol Immunotoxicol* 14(1–2):63–77, 1992.

55. Matthies H; Staak S; Krug M: Fucose and fucosyllactose enhance in-vitro hippocampal long-term potentiation. *Brain Res* 725(2): 276–280, 1996.

56. Nogami M; Tsuji Y; Kubo M; et al.: Studies on *Ganoderma lucidum*. VI. Anti-allergic effect. (1). *Yakugaku Zasshi* 106(7):594–599, 1986.

57. Cherian L; Klemm WR: Ethanol effects on total sialic acid of various brain regions and visceral organs. *Alcohol* 8:389–393, 1991.

58. Cherian L; Mathew J; Klemm WR: Ethanol-induced hydrolysis of brain sialoglycoconjugates in the rat: *Alcohol Clin Exp Res* 13(3): 435–438, 1989.

59. Gilmore N; Cherian L; Klemm WR: Ganglioside or sialic acid attenuates ethanol-induced decrements in locomotion, nose-poke exploration, and anxiety, but not body temperature. *Prog Neuro-Psychopharmacol Biol Psychiatr* 15:91–104, 1991.

60. Klemm WR; Boyles R; Mathew J; Cherian L: Gangliosides, or sialic acid, antagonize ethanol intoxication. *Life Sci* 43:1837–1843, 1988.

61. Berg D; Berg LH; Couvaras J; Harrison H: Chronic fatigue syndrome and/or fibromyalgia as a variation of antiphospholipid antibody syndrome: an explanatory model and approach to laboratory diagnosis. *Blood Coagul Fibrinolysis* 10(7):435–438, 1999.

62. Zhao Y: Inhibitory effects of alcoholic extract of *Cordyceps sinensis* on abdominal aortic thrombus formation in rabbits. *Chung Hua I Hsueh Tsa Chih* 71(11):612–615, 42, 1991.

63. Veldman FJ; Nair CH; Vorster HH; et al.: Possible mechanisms through which dietary pectin influences fibrin network architecture in hypercholesterolaemic subjects. *Throm Res* 93(6):253–264, 1999.

64. Vercoulen JH; Swanink CM; Fennis JF; et al.: Prognosis in chronic fatigue syndrome: A prospective study on the natural course. *J Neurol Neurosurg Psychiatry* 60(5):489–494, 1996.

65. Mays P: CDC diverts chronic fatigue funds. Associated Press, July 6, 1999.

66. Strauss V: GAO to probe diversion of CDC research funds audit: Money for chronic fatigue study used elsewhere. *Washington Post,* July 21, 1999, p. A19.

## 10 MANAGING ARTHRITIS, DIABETES, AND OTHER CHRONIC ILLNESSES

1. Appleton J: Glucosamine and chondroitin in the treatment of osteoarthritis. *Nutr Res Rev* Summer:134, 2000.

2. Deal CL; Moskowitz RW: Nutraceuticals as therapeutic agents in osteoarthritis. The role of glucosamine, chondroitin sulfate and collagen hydrolysate. *Rheum Dis Clin North Am* 25(2):379–395, 1999.

3. Setnikar I; Cereda R; Pacini MA; Revel L: Antireactive properties of glucosamine sulfate. *Arzneimittelforschung* 41(2):157–161, 1991.

4. Debi R; Robinson D; Agar G; et al.: GAG for osteoarthritis of the knee—a prospective study. *Harefuah* 138(6):451–453, 518, 2000.

5. Brody J: Personal health, *New York Times,* Jan 15, 1997.

6. Bond A; Alavi A; Axford JS; et al.: A detailed lectin analysis of IgG glycosylation, demonstrating disease specific changes in terminal galactose and N-acetylglucosamine. *J Autoimmun* 10(1):77–85, 1997.

7. Kötz K; Hänsler M; Sauer H; et al.: Immunoglobulin G galactosylation deficiency determined by isoelectric focusing and lectin affinoblotting in differential diagnosis of rheumatoid arthritis. *Electrophoresis* 17(3):533–534, 1996.

8. Davis RH; Stewart GJ; Bregman PJ: *Aloe vera* and the inflamed synovial pouch model. *J Am Podiatr Med Assoc* 82(3):140–148, 1992.

9. Saito H; Ishiguro T; Imanishi K; Suzuki I: Pharmacological studies on plant lectin aloctin A. II. Inhibitory effect of aloctin A on experi-

mental models of inflammation in rats. *Jpn J Pharmacol* 32(1): 139–142, 1982.

10. Davis RH; Maro NP: *Aloe vera* and gibberellin. Anti-inflammatory activity in diabetes. *J Am Podiatr Med Assoc* 79(1):24–26, 1989.

11. Ghannam N; Kingston M; Al-Meshaal IA; et al.: The antidiabetic activity of aloes: Preliminary clinical and experimental observations. *Horm Res* 24(4):288–294, 1986.

12. Bunyapraphatsara N; Yongchaiyudha S; Rungpitarasangsi V; Chokechaijaroenporn O: Antidiabetic activity of *Aloe vera* L. juice II. Clinical trial in diabetes mellitus patients in combination with glibenclamide. *Phytomedicine* 3(3):245–248, 1996.

13. Yuan Z; He P; Cui J; Takeuchi H: Hypoglycemic effect of water-soluble polysaccharide from Auricularia auricula-judae Quel. on genetically diabetic KK-Aʸ mice. *Biosci Biotechnol Biochem* 62(10): 1898–1903, 1998.

14. Hikino H; Mizuno T: Hypoglycemic actions of some heteroglycans of *Ganoderma lucidum* fruit bodies. *Planta Med* 55(4):385, 1989.

15. Kiho T; Ookubo K; Usui S; et al.: Structural features and hypoglycemic activity of a polysaccharide (CS-F10) from the cultured mycelium of *Cordyceps sinensis*. *Biol Pharm Bull* 22(9):968, 1999.

16. Kubo K; Aoki H; Nanba H: Anti-diabetic activity present in the fruit body of *Grifola frondosa* (Maitake). I. *Biol Pharm Bull* 17(8): 1106–1110, 1994.

17. Koo MWL: *Aloe vera:* Antiulcer and antidiabetic effects. *Phytotherapy Res* 8:461–464, 1994.

18. van der Hem LG; van der Vliet JA; Bocken CF; et al.: Ling zhi-8: Studies of a new immunomodulating agent. *Transplantation* 60(5): 438–443, 1995.

19. Kiho, Ookubo, Usui, et al., pp. 966–970.

20. Kiho T; Yamane A; Hui J; et al.: Polysaccharides in fungi. XXXVI. Hypoglycemic activity of a polysaccharide (CS-F30) from the cultural mycelium of *Cordyceps sinensis* and its effect on glucose in mouse liver. *Biol Pharm Bull* 19(2):294–296, 1996.

21. Murch SH; MacDonald TT; Walker-Smith JA; et al.: Disruption of sulphated glycosaminoglycans in intestinal inflammation. *Lancet* 341(8847):711–714, 1993.

22. Russell AL: Glycosaminoglycan (GAG) deficiency in protective barrier as an underlying primary cause of ulcerative colitis, Crohn's disease, interstitial cystitis and possibly Reiter's syndrome. *Med Hypotheses* 52(4):297–301, 1999.

23. Russell.

24. Russell.

25. Parsons CL; Boychuk D; Jones S; et al.: Bladder surface gly-cosaminoglycans: An epithelial permeability barrier. *J Urol* 143(1): 139–142, 1990.

26. Russell, pp. 297–300.

27. Moore N: *The Missing Link.* Seattle, WA: Validation Press, 1999, p. 233.

28. Clamp JR; Fraser G; Read AE: Study of the carbohydrate content of mucus glycoproteins from normal and diseased colons. *Clin Sci (Colch)* 61(2):229–234, 1981.

29. Moore, p. 232.

30. Reynolds T; Dweck AC: *Aloe vera* leaf gel: A review update. *J Ethnopharmacol* 68(1-3):15, 1999.

31. Kelly GS: Larch arabinogalactan: Clinical relevance of a novel immune-enhancing polysaccharide. *Altern Med Rev* 4(2):96–103, 1999.

32. Yang LY; Chen A; Kuo YC; Lin CY: Efficacy of a pure compound H1-A extracted from *Cordyceps sinensis* on autoimmune disease of MRL lpr/lpr mice. *J Lab Clin Med* 134(5):492–500, 1999.

33. Guan YJ; Hu Z; Hou M: Effect of *Cordyceps sinensis* on T-lymphocyte subsets in chronic renal failure. *Chung Kuo Chung His I Chieh Ho Tsa Chih* 12(6):338–339, 323, 1992.

34. Zhu JS; Halpern GM; Jones K: The scientific rediscovery of a precious ancient Chinese herbal regimen: *Cordyceps sinensis.* Part II. *J Alt Complement Med* 4(4):433, 1998.

35. Li LS; Zheng F; Liu ZH: Experimental study on effect of *Cordyceps sinensis* in ameliorating aminoglycoside-induced nephrotoxicity. *Chung Kuo Chung His I Chieh Ho Tsa Chih* 16(12):733–737, 1996.

36. Zhen F; Tian J; Li LS: Mechanism and therapeutic effect of *Cordyceps sinensis* (CS) on aminoglycoside induced acute renal failure (ARF) in rats. *Chung Kuo Chung Hsi I Chieh Ho Tsa Chih* 12(5): 288–291, 262, 1992.

37. Xu F; Huang JB; Jiang L; et al.: Amelioration of cyclosporin nephrotoxicity by *Cordyceps sinensis* in kidney-transplanted recipients [letter]. *Nephrol Dial Transplant* 10(1):142–143, 1995.

38. van der Hem, van der Vliet, Bocken, pp. 438–443.

## 11 INHIBITING CANCER

1. Kidd P: The use of mushroom glucans and proteoglycans in cancer treatment. *Altern Med Rev* 5(1):16, 2000.
2. Kidd, p. 8.
3. Nanba H; Kubo K: Effect of maitake D-fraction on cancer prevention. *Ann N Y Acad Sci* 833:204–207, 1997.
4. Nanba H: Activity of maitake D-fraction to inhibit carcinogenesis and metastasis. *Ann N Y Acad Sci* 768:243–245, 1995.
5. Matsuo T; Kurahashi Y; Nishida S; et al.: Granulopoietic effects of lentinan in mice: Effects on GM-CFC and 5-FU-induced leukopenia. *Gan To Kagaku Ryoho* 14(5, pt. 1):1310–1314, 1987.
6. Hsu HY; Lian SL; Lin CC: Radioprotective effect of *Ganoderma lucidum* (Leyss. ex. Fr.) Karst after X-ray irradiation in mice. *Am J Chin Med* 18(1-2):61–69, 1990.
7. Pande S; Kumar M; Kumar A: Radioprotective efficacy of *Aloe vera* leaf extract. *Pharmaceut Biol* 36(3):227–232, 1998.
8. Egger SF; Brown GS; Kelsey LS; et al.: Hematopoietic augmentation by a beta-(1,4)-linked mannan. *Cancer Immunol Immunother* 43(4): 195–205, 1996.
9. Roberts DB; Travis EL: Acemannan-containing wound dressing gel reduces radiation-induced skin reactions in C3H mice. *Int J Radiat Oncol Biol Phys* 32(4):1047–1052, 1995.
10. Kurashige S; Akuzawa Y; Endo F: Effects of *Lentinus edodes; Grifola frondosa* and *Pleurotus ostreatus* administration on cancer outbreak, and activities of macrophages and lymphocytes in mice treated with a carcinogen, N-butyl-N-butanolnitrosamine. *Immunopharmacol Immunotoxicol* 19(2):175–183, 1997.
11. Mizutani Y; Yoshida O: Activation by the protein-bound polysaccharide PSK (krestin) of cytotoxic lymphocytes that act on fresh autologous tumor cells and T24 human urinary bladder transitional carcinoma cell line in patients with urinary bladder cancer. *J Urol* 145(5):1082–1087, 1991.
12. Mickey DD: Combined therapeutic effects of an immunomodulator, PSK, and chemotherapy with carboquone on rat bladder carcinoma. *Cancer Chemother Pharmacol* 15(1):54–58, 1985.
13. Yokoe T; Iino Y; Takei H: HLA antigen as predictive index for the outcome of breast cancer patients with adjuvant immunochemotherapy with PSK. *Anticancer Res* 17(4A):2815–2818, 1997.
14. Fujii T; Saito K; Oguchi Y; et al.: Effects of the protein-bound

polysaccharide preparation PSK on spontaneous breast cancer in mice. *J Int Med Res* 16(4):286–293, 1988.

15. Iino Y; Takai Y; Sugamata N; Morishita Y: PSK (krestin) potentiates chemotherapeutic effects of tamoxifen on rat mammary carcinomas. *Anticancer Res* 12(6B):2101–2103, 1992.

16. Nanba, Kubo, pp. 204–207.

17. Torisu M; Hayashi Y; Ishimitsu T; et al.: Significant prolongation of disease-free period gained by oral polysaccharide K (PSK) administration after curative surgical operation of colorectal cancer. *Cancer Immunol Immunother* 31(5):261–268, 1990.

18. Torisu, Hayashi, Ishimitsu.

19. Kidd, pp. 4–27.

20. Borchers AT; Stern JS; Hackman RM; et al.: Mushrooms, tumors and immunity. *Proc Soc Exp Biol Med* 221:287, 1999.

21. Taguchi T: Clinical efficacy of lentinan on patients with stomach cancer: End point results of a four-year follow-up survey. *Cancer Detect Prev Suppl* 1:333–349, 1987.

22. Taguchi T: Effects of lentinan in advanced or recurrent cases of gastric, colorectal, and breast cancer. *Gan To Kagaku Ryoho* 10(2, pt. 2):387–393, 1983.

23. Ogoshi K; Satou H; Isono K; et al.: Possible predictive markers of immunotherapy in esophageal cancer: Retrospective analysis of a randomized study. *Cancer Invest* 13:363–369, 1995.

24. Nagao T; Komatsuda M; Yamauchi K; et al.: Chemoimmunotherapy with krestin in acute leukemia. *Tokai J Exp Clin Med* 6(2):141–146, 1981.

25. Kidd, pp. 6–7.

26. Suto T; Fukuda S; Moriya N; et al.: Clinical study of biological response modifiers as maintenance therapy for hepatocellular carcinoma. *Cancer Chemother Pharmacol* 33(suppl):S145–148, 1994.

27. Nanba, pp. 243–245.

28. Nanba.

29. Nanba, Kubo, pp. 204–207.

30. Shiga J; Maruyama T; Takahashi H; et al.: Effect of PSK, a protein-bound polysaccharide preparation, on liver tumors of Syrian hamsters induced by Thorotrast injection. *Acta Pathol Jpn* 43(9):475–480, 1993.

31. Hayakawa K; Mitsuhashi N; Saito Y; et al.: Effect of krestin as adjuvant treatment following radical radiotherapy in non-small cell lung cancer patients. *Cancer Detect Prev* 21(1):71–77, 1997.

32. Yefenof E; Gafanovitch I; Oron E; et al.: Prophylactic intervention in radiation-leukemia-virus-induced murine lymphoma by the biological response modifier polysaccharide K. *Cancer Immunol Immunother* 41(6):389–396, 1995.

33. Yefenof E; Einat E; Klein E: Potentiation of T cell immunity against radiation-leukemia-virus-induced lymphoma by polysaccharide K. *Cancer Immunol Immunother* 34(2):133–137, 1991.

34. Go P; Chung CH: Adjuvant PSK immunotherapy in patients with carcinoma of the nasopharynx. *J Int Med Res* 17(2):141–149, 1989.

35. Chung CH; Go P; Chang KH: PSK immunotherapy in cancer patients—a preliminary report. *Chun Hua Min Kuo Wei Sheng Wu Chi Mien I Hsueh Tsa Chih* 20(3):210–216, 1987.

36. Ghoneum M; Jewettt A: Production of tumor necrosis factor-alpha and interferon-gamma from human peripheral blood lymphocytes by MGN-3, a modified arabinoxylan from rice bran, and its synergy with interleukin-2 in vitro. *Cancer Detect Prev* 24(4):314–324, 2000.

37. Mickey DD; Bencuya PS; Foulkes K: Effects of the immunomodulator PSK on growth of human prostate adenocarcinoma in immunodeficient mice. *Int J Immunopharmacol* 11(7):829–838, 1989.

38. Xu R; Peng X; Chen GZ; Chen GL: Effects of *Cordyceps sinensis* on natural killer activity and colony formation of $B_{16}$ melanoma. *Chin Med J* 104(1):97–101, 1992.

39. Adachi K; Nanba H; Kuroda H: Potentiation of host-mediated antitumor activity in mice by β-glucan obtained from *Grifola frondosa* (maitake). *Chem Pharm Bull* 35(1): 262–270, 1987.

40. Hauer J; Anderer FA: Mechanism of stimulation of human natural killer cytotoxicity by arabinogalactan from *Larix occidentalis*. *Cancer Immunol Immunother* 36(4):237–244, 1993.

41. Liu C; Lu S; Ji MR: Effects of *Cordyceps sinensis* (CS) on in vitro natural killer cells. *Chung Kuo Chung Hsi I Chieh Ho Tsa Chih* 12(5): 267–269, 259, 1992.

42. Mickey DD; Carvalho L; Foulkes K: Combined therapeutic effects of conventional agents and an immunomodulator, polysaccharide K, on rat prostatic adenocarcinoma. *J Urol* 142(6):1594–1598, 1989.

43. Pienta KJ; Naik H; Akhtar A; et al.: Inhibition of spontaneous metastasis in a rat prostate cancer model by oral administration of modified citrus pectin. *J Natl Cancer Inst* 87(5):348–353, 1995.

44. Fullerton SA; Samadi AA; Tortorelis DG; et al.: Induction of apoptosis in human prostatic cancer cells with beta-glucan. *Mol Urol* 4(1): 7–14, 2000.

45. Harris C; Pierce K; King G; et al.: Efficacy of acemannan in treatment of canine and feline spontaneous neoplasms. *Mol Biother* 3(4):207–213, 1991.

46. Maruyama H; Yamazaki K; Murofushi S; et al.: Antitumor activity of *Sarcodon aspratus* (Berk.) *S. ito* and *Ganoderma lucidum* (Fr.) Karst. *J Pharmacobiodyn* 12(2):118–123, 1989.

47. Wang G; Zhang J; Mizuno T; et al.: Antitumor active polysaccharides from the Chinese mushroom Songshan lingzhi, the fruiting body of *Ganoderma tsugae. Biosci Biotechnol Biochem* 57(6):894–900, 1993.

48. Zhang J; Wang G; Li H; et al.: Antitumor active protein-containing glycans from the Chinese mushroom Songshan lingzhi; *Ganoderma tsugae* mycelium. *Biosci Biotechnol Biochem* 58(7):1202–1205, 1994.

49. Ebina T; Fujimiya Y: Antitumor effect of a peptide-glucan preparation extracted from *Agaricus blazei* in a double-grafted tumor system in mice. *Biotherapy* 11(4):259–265, 1998.

50. Ralamboranto L; Rakotovao LH; Le Deaut JY; et al.: Immunomodulating properties of an extract isolated and partially purified from *Aloe vahombe*. 3. Study of antitumoral properties and contribution to the chemical nature and active principle. *Arch Inst Pasteur Madagascar* 50(1):227–256, 1982.

51. Matsunaga K; Ohhara M; Oguchi Y; et al.: Antimetastatic effect of PSK, a protein-bound polysaccharide, against the B16-BL6 mouse melanoma. *Invasion Metastasis* 16(1):27–38, 1996.

52. Matsunaga K; Aota M; Nyunoya Y; et al.: Antitumor effect of biological response modifier, PSK, on C57BL/6 mice with syngeneic melanoma B16 and its mode of action. *Oncology* 51(4):303–308, 1994.

53. Ishihara Y; Fujii T; Iijima H; et al.: The role of neutrophils as cytotoxic cells in lung metastasis: Suppression of tumor cell metastasis by a biological response modifier (PSK). *In Vivo* 12(2):175–182, 1998.

54. Matsunaga, Ohhara, Oguchi, et al.

55. Li Y; Chen G; Jiang D: Effect of *Cordyceps sinesis* on erythropoiesis in mouse bone marrow. *Chin Med J* 106(4):313–316, 1993.

56. Nakazato H; Koike A; Saji S; et al.: Efficacy of immunochemotherapy as adjuvant treatment after curative resection of gastric cancer. *Lancet* 343:1122–1126, 1994.

57. Takeshita M: Nonspecific cell-mediated immunity in gastric cancer patients—with special reference to immuno-reactivity of the re-

gional lymph node and preoperative immunotherapy. *Nippon Geka Gakkai Zasshi* 84(8):679–691, 1983.

58. Takeshita M; Kobori T; Sudo E; et al.: Preoperative immunotherapy for gastric cancer patients—immunomodulating effect of levamisole and lentinan on cell-mediated immunity and regional lymph node. *Gan To Kagaku Ryoho* 9(6):1052–1060, 1982.

59. Kondo M; Torisu M: Evaluation of an anticancer activity of a protein-bound polysaccharide PSK (krestin). In Torisu M, Yoshida T, eds. *Basic Mechanisms and Clinical Treatment of Tumor Metastasis.* New York: Academic Press, 1985, pp. 623–636.

60. Kidd, pp. 16–18.

61. Romano CF; Lipton A; Harvey HA; et al.: A phase II study of Catrix-S in solid tumors. *J Biol Response Mod* 4(6):585–589, 1985.

62. Puccio C; Mittelman A; Chun H; et al.: Treatment of metastatic renal cell carcinoma with Catrix. *Proc Annu Meet Am Soc Clin Oncol* 13:A769, 1994.

63. Lissoni P; Giani L; Zerbini S; et al.: Biotherapy with the pineal immunomodulating hormone melatonin versus melatonin plus *Aloe vera* in untreatable advanced solid neoplasms. *Nat Immun* 16(1): 27–33, 1998.

## 12 FIGHTING HEPATITIS, HIV, AND OPPORTUNISTIC INFECTIONS

1. Weiss Harry C: Hepatitis C sucks. *Indianapolis Monthly,* June 2000, pp. 94–95, 173–175.

2. Zhu JS; Halpern GM; Jones K: The scientific rediscovery of a precious ancient Chinese herbal medicine: *Cordyceps sinensis.* Part II. *J Altern Complement Med* 4(4):441–442, 1998.

3. Zhu JL; Liu C: Modulating effects of extractum semen Persicae and cultivated *Cordyceps hyphae* on immunodysfunction of inpatients with posthepatic cirrhosis. *Chung Kuo Chung Hsi I Chieh Ho Tsa Chih* 12(4):207–209, 195, 1992.

4. Zhou L; Yang W; Xu Y; et al.: Short-term curative effect of cultured *Cordyceps sinensis* (Berk.) Sacc. Mycelia in chronic hepatitis B. *Chung Kuo Chung Yao Tsa Chih* 15(1):53–55, 65, 1990.

5. Zhu JS; Halpern GM; Jones K: The scientific rediscovery of an ancient Chinese herbal medicine: *Cordyceps sinensis.* Part I. *J Altern Complement Med* 4(3):293, 1998.

6. Jong SC; Birmingham JM: Medicinal benefits of the mushroom *Ganoderma. Adv Appl Microbiol* 37:114, 1992.

7. Liu G; Bao T; Wei H; Song Z: Some pharmacological actions of *Ganoderma lucidum* and *G. japonicum* (FR) *Llyod* on mouse liver. *Yao Hseuh Hseuh Pao* 14(5):287, 1979.

8. Liu G; Wang G; Wei H; et al.: A comparison of the protective actions of biphenyl dimethyl-dicarboxylate, trans-stilbene, alcoholic extracts of Fructus Schizandrae and *Ganoderma* against experimental liver injury in mice. *Yao Hseuh Hseuh Pao* 14(10):14, 1979.

9. Jones K: Maitake: A potent medicinal food. *Altern Complement Ther,* Dec 1998, pp. 420–429.

10. Kidd P: The use of mushroom glucans and proteoglycans in cancer treatment. *Altern Med Rev* 5(1):7, 2000.

11. Shilts R: *And the Band Played On: Politics, People and the AIDS Epidemic.* New York: St. Martin's Press, 2000 (paperback).

12. Genentech Connection: Current Seminar. URL: http://www.accessexcellence.com/LC/SS/ed_connection.html.

13. Gordon M; Bihari B; Goosby E; et al.: A placebo-controlled trial of the immune modulator lentinan in HIV-positive patients: A phase I/II trial. *J Med* 29(5-6):305–330, 1998.

14. Gordon M; Guralnik M; Kaneko Y; et al.: A phase II controlled study of a combination of the immune modulator lentinan with didanosine (ddI) in HIV patients with CD4 cells of 200–500/mm$^3$. *J Med* 26(5-6):193–207, 1995.

15. Cichoke A: Maitake—The king of mushrooms. *Townsend Letter for Doctors,* May 1994, p. 432.

16. Montaner JS; Gill J; Singer J; et al.: Double-blind placebo-controlled pilot trial of acemannan in advanced human immunodeficiency virus disease. *J Acquir Immune Defic Syndr Hum Retrovirol* 12(2): 153–157, 1996.

17. Sheets MA; Unger BA; Giggleman GF; Tizard IR: Studies of the effect of acemannan on retrovirus infections: Clinical stabilization of feline leukemia virus-infected cats. *Mol Biother* 3(1):41–45, 1991.

18. Kahlon JB; Kemp MC; Yawei N; et al.: In vitro evaluation of the synergistic antiviral effects of acemannan in combination with azidothymidine and acyclovir. *Mol Biother* 3(4):214–223, 1991.

19. Kim HS; Kacew S; Lee BM: In vitro chemopreventive effects of plant polysaccharides *(Aloe barbadensis miller, Lentinus edodes, Ganoderma lucidum* and *Coriolus versicolor). Carcinogenesis* 20(8):1637–1640, 1999.

20. Sabeh F; Wright T; Norton SJ: Purification and characterization of a

glutathione peroxidase from the *Aloe vera* plant. *Enzyme Protein* 47(2):92–98, 1993.

21. Pang ZJ; Chen Y; Zhou M; Wan J: Effect of polysaccharide krestin on glutathione peroxidase gene expression in mouse peritoneal macrophages. *Br J Biomed Sci* 57(2):130–136, 2000.

22. Ando T; Motokawa I; Sakurai K; et al.: Effects of PSK on resistance to bacterial infection in splenectomized mice. *Oncology* 45(3): 224–229, 1988.

23. Sabolovic D; Galoppin L: Effect of a protein bound polysaccharide (PSK) on tumor development and infections in splenectomized rats and mice. *Int J Immunopharmacol* 8(1):41–46, 1986.

24. Ando T; Motokawa I; Sakurai K; et al.: Influence of PSK (krestin) on resistance to infection of Pseudomonas aeroginosa in tumor-bearing mice. *Cancer Chemother Pharmacol* 20(3):198–202, 1987.

25. Stepinska M; Trafny EA: Modulation of Pseudomonas aeruginosa adherence to collagen type I and type II by carbohydrates. *FEMS Immunol Med Microbiol* 12(3–4):187–194, 1995.

26. Barghouthi S; Guerdoud LM; Speert DP: Inhibition by dextran of Pseudomonas aeroginosa adherence to epithelial cells. *Am J Respir Crit Care Med* 154(6, pt. 1):1788–1793, 1996.

27. Azghani AO; Williams I; Holiday DB; Johnson AR: A beta-linked mannan inhibits adherence of *Pseudomonas aeruginosa* to human lung epithelial cells. *Glycobiology* 5(1):39–44, 1995.

28. Bao ZD; Wu ZG; Zheng F: Amelioration of aminoglycoside nephrotoxicity by *Cordyceps sinensis* in old patients. *Chung Kuo Chung Hsi I Chieh Ho Tsa Chih* 14(5):271–273, 259, 1994.

## 13   GLYCONUTRIENTS AS PREVENTIVE MEDICINE

1. Krause D; Mastro AM; Handte G; et al.: Immune function did not decline with aging in apparently healthy, well-nourished women. *Mech Ageing Dev* 112(1):43–57, 1999.

2. Kawakami K; Kadota J; Iida K; et al.: Reduced immune function and malnutrition in the elderly. *Tohoku J Exp Med* 187(2):157–171, 1999.

3. Zhu JS; Halpern GM; Jones K: The scientific rediscovery of an ancient Chinese herbal medicine: *Cordyceps sinensis*. Part I. *J Altern Complement Med* 4(3):295–296, 1998.

4. Zhang ZJ; Luo HL; Li JS: Clinical and experimental studies on elimination of oxygen free radical of jinshuibao capsule in treating senile deficiency syndrome and its deoxyribonucleic acid damage

repairing effects. *Chung Kuo Chung Hsi I Chieh Ho Tsa Chih* 17(1): 35–38, 1997.

5. Lei LS; Lin ZB: Effects of *Ganoderma* polysaccharides on the activity of DNA polymerase alpha of splenocytes and immune function in aged mice. *Yao Hsueh Hsueh Pao* 28(8):577–582, 1993.

6. Jones K: Reishi mushroom: Ancient medicine in modern times. *Altern Complement Ther,* Aug 1998, p. 258.

7. Jones.

8. Zhu, Halpern, Jones, pp. 297–298.

9. Zhu, Halpern, Jones, pp. 298–299.

10. Zhu, Halpern, Jones, p. 297.

11. Zhu, Halpern, Jones, p. 297.

12. Beers MH; Berkow R (eds): *The Merck Manual: Diagnosis and Therapy.* 17th Ed (Centennial Edition). Whitehouse Station, NJ: Merck, 1999, p. 58.

13. Jones K: Maitake: A potent medicinal food. *Altern Complement Ther,* Dec 1998, p. 422.

14. Kaats GR; Keith SC; Croft HA; et al.: Dietary supplements and a behavior modification plan improve the safety and efficacy of pharmacotherapy. *Adv Ther* 15(3):167–179, 1998.

15. Kubo K; Nanba H: The effect of maitake mushrooms on liver and serum lipids. *Altern Ther* 2(5):62–66, 1996.

16. Lee CK; Han SS; Mo YK; et al.: Prevention of ultraviolet radiation-induced suppression of accessory cell function of Langerhans cells by *Aloe vera* gel components. *Immunopharmacology* 37(2-3):153–162, 1997.

17. Roberts DB; Travis EL: Acemannan-containing wound dressing gel reduces radiation-induced skin reactions in C3H mice. *Int J Radiat Oncol Biol Phys* 32(4):1047–1052, 1995.

18. Strickland FM; Pelley RP; Kripke ML: Prevention of ultraviolet radiation-induced suppression of contact and delayed hypersensitivity by Aloe barbadensis gel extract. *J Invest Dermatol* 102(2): 197–204, 1994.

19. Byeon SW; Pelley RP; Ullrich SE; Waller TA; Bucana CD; Strickland FM: Aloe barbadensis extracts reduce the production of interleukin-10 after exposure to ultraviolet radiation. *J Invest Dermatol* 110(5):811–817, 1998.

20. Nishizake Y; Yoshizane C; Toshimori Y; et al.: Disaccharide-trehalose inhibits bone resorption in ovariectomized mice. *Nutrition Res* 20(5):654, 2000.

21. Nishizake, Yoshizane, Toshimori, pp. 653–664.

22. Kodama T; Reddy VN; Giblin F; et al.: Scanning electron microscopy of X-ray-induced cataract in mice on normal and galactose diet. *Ophthalmic Res* 15(6):324–333, 1983.
23. Taura T; Giblin FJ; Reddy VN: Further observations of the effect of galactose on the development of X-ray-induced cataract in mice. *Exp Eye Res* 41(4):527–543, 1985.

## 14  WORKING WITH MEMORY, INSOMNIA, ANXIETY, DEPRESSION, AND ADHD

1. Zanetta JP: Structure and functions of lectins in the central and peripheral nervous system. *Acta Anat (Basel)* 161(1-4):180–195, 1998.
2. Zhou D; Chen C; Jiang S; et al.: Expression of beta 1,4-galacosyltransferase in the development of the mouse brain. *Biochem Biophys Acta* 1425(1):204–208, 1998.
3. Dupree JL; Suzuki K; Popko B: Galactolipids in the formation and function of the myelin sheath. *Microsc Res Tech* 41(5):431–440, 1998.
4. Newman PE: Alzheimer's disease revisited. *Med Hypotheses* 54(5): 774–776, 2000.
5. Youdim KA; Martin A; Joseph JA: Essential fatty acids and the brain: Possible health implications. *Int J Dev Neurosci* 18(4-5):383–399, 2000.
6. Bennett CN; Horrobin DF: Gene targets related to phospholipid and fatty acid metabolism in schizophrenia and other psychiatric disorders: An update. *Prostaglandins Leukot Essent Fatty Acids* 63(1-2): 47–59, 2000.
7. Horrobin DF; Bennett CN: Depression and bipolar disorder: relationships to impaired fatty acid and phospholipid metabolism and to diabetes, cardiovascular disease, immunological abnormalities, cancer, ageing and osteoporosis. Possible candidate genes. *Prostaglandins Leukot Essent Fatty Acids* 60(4):217–234, 1999.
8. Gallai V; Sarchielli P; Trequattrini A; et al.: Cytokine secretion and eicosanoid production in the peripheral blood mononuclear cells of MS patients undergoing dietary supplementation with n-3 polyunsaturated fatty acids. *J Neuroimmunol* 56(2):143–153, 1995.
9. Bates D: Dietary lipids and multiple sclerosis. *Ups J Med Sci Suppl* 48:173–187, 1990.
10. Freeman MP: Omega-3 fatty acids in psychiatry: A review. *Ann Clin Psychiatry* 12(3):159–165, 2000.
11. Matthies H Jr; Kretlow J; Matthies H; et al.: Glycosylation of proteins

during a critical time window is necessary for the maintenance of long-term potentiation in the hippocampal CA1 region. *Neuroscience* 91(1):175–183, 1999.

12. Matthies H; Staak S; Krug M: Fucose and fucosyllactose enhance in-vitro hippocampal long-term potentiation. *Brain Res* 725(2): 276–280, 1996.

13. Dunn AJ; Hogan EL: Brain gangliosides: Increased incorporation of (1-³H) glucosamine during training. *Pharmacol Biochem Behav* 3:605–612, 1975.

14. Perlmutter D: Functional therapeutics in neurodegenerative disease. *J Applied Nutr* 51(1):4, 1999.

15. Hobbs C: *Medicinal Mushrooms: An Exploration of Tradition, Healing, and Culture.* Santa Cruz, CA: Botanica Press, 1995, p. 103.

16. Honda K; Komoda Y; Inoue S: Sleep-promoting effects of *Ganoderma* extracts in rats: Comparison between long-term and acute administrations. *Tokyo Ika Shika Daigaku Iyo Kizai Kenkuyusho Hokoku* 22:77–82, 1988.

17. Jones K: Reishi mushroom: Ancient medicine in modern times. *Altern Complement Therapies,* Aug 1998, p. 256.

18. Waldman ID; Rowe DC; Abramowitz A; et al.: Association and linkage of the dopamine transporter gene and attention-deficit hyperactivity disorder in children: Heterogeneity owing to diagnostic subtype and severity. *Am J Hum Genetics* 63(6):1767–1776, 1998.

19. Faraone SV; Biederman J: Neurobiology of attention-deficit hyperactivity disorder. *Biol Psychiatry* 44(10):951–958, 1998.

20. Krummel DA; Seligson FH; Guthrie HA: Hyperactivity: Is candy causal? *Crit Rev Food Sci Nutr* 36(1-2):31–47, 1996.

21. Morgan BLG; Winick M: Effects of environmental stimulation on brain N-acetylneuraminic acid content and behavior. *J Nutr* 110(3): 425–432, 1980.

22. Backstrom JR; Westphal RS; Canton H; Sanders-Bush E: Identification of rat serotonin 5-HT2C receptors as glycoproteins containing N-linked oligosaccharides. *Brain Res Mol* 33(2):311–318, 1995.

23. Abramowski D; Staufenbiel M: Identification of the 5-hydroxytryptamine 2C receptor as a 60-kDa N-glycosylated protein in choroid plexus and hippocampus. *J Neurochem* 65(2):782–790, 1995.

24. Rao ML; Hawellek B; Papassotiropoulos A; et al.: Upregulation of the platelet serotonin 2A receptor and low serotonin in suicidal psychiatric patients. *Neuropsychobiology* 38(2):84–89, 1998.

25. Hurwitz TA; Clark C; Murphy E; et al.: Regional cerebral glucose

metabolism in major depressive disorder. *Can J Psychiatry* 35(8): 684–688, 1990.

26. Drevets WC; Ongur D; Price JL: Reduced glucose metabolism in the subgenual prefrontal cortex in unipolar depression. *Mol Psychiatry* 3(3):190–191, 1998.

27. Delvenne V; Goldman S; Simon Y; et al.: Brain hypometabolism of glucose in bulimia nervosa. *Int J Eat Disord* 21(4):313–320, 1997.

28. Delvenne V; Lostra F; Goldman S; et al.: Brain hypometabolism of glucose in anorexia nervosa: A PET scan study. *Bio Psychiatry* 37(3):161–169, 1995.

29. Baxter LR Jr.: Positron emission tomography studies of cerebral glucose meabolism in obsessive-compulsive disorder. *J Clin Psychiatry* 55(suppl):54–59, 1994.

30. Holden RJ: The role of brain insulin in the neurophysiology of serious mental disorders: Review. *Med Hypotheses* 52(3):193–200, 1999.

31. Cassidy F; Ahearn E; Carroll BJ: Elevated frequency of diabetes mellitus in hospitalized manic-depressive patients. *Am J Psychiatry* 156(9):1417–1420, 1999.

32. Baxter LR Jr; Schwartz JM; Phelps ME; et al.: Reduction of prefrontal cortex glucose metabolism common to three types of depression. *Arch Gen Psychiatry* 46(3):243–250, 1989.

33. Svanborg P; Mattila-Evenden M; Gustavsson PJ; et al.: Associations between plasma glucose and DSM-III-R cluster B personality traits in psychiatric outpatients. *Neuropsychobiology* 41(2):79–87, 2000.

34. Holden, pp. 193–200.

## 15 REVERSING HEART DISEASE

1. Alvarez J; Cremniter D; Gluck N; et al.: Low serum cholesterol in violent but not in non-violent suicide attempters. *Psychiatry Res* 95(2):103–108, 2000.

2. Abbott C; Meadows AB; Lier K: Low cholesterol and noncardiovascular mortality. *Mil Med* 1165(6):466–469, 2000.

3. Davidson M; Kuo CC; Middaugh JP; et al.: Confirmed previous infection with Chlamydia pneumonia (TWAR) and its presence in early coronary atherosclerosis. *Circulation* 98(7):628–633, 1998.

4. Liu SX; Zhou M; Chen Y; et al.: Lipoperoxidative injury to macrophages by oxidatively modified low-density lipoprotein may play an important role in foam cell formation. *Atherosclerosis* 121(1):55–61, 1996.

5. Blum A; Miller HI: The role of inflammation in atherosclerosis. *Isr J Med Sci* 32(11):1059–1065, 1996.

6. Sabeh F; Wright T; Norton SJ: Purification and characterization of glutathione peroxidase from the *Aloe vera* plant. *Enzyme Protein* 47(2):92–98, 1993.

7. Pang ZJ; Chen Y; Zhou M; Wan J: Effect of polysaccharide krestin on glutathione peroxidase gene expression in mouse peritoneal macrophages. *Br J Biomed Sci* 57(2):130–136, 2000.

8. Kim HS; Kacew S; Lee BM: In vitro chemopreventive effects of plant polysaccharides *(Aloe bearbadensis miller, Lentinus edodes, Ganoderma lucidum and Coriolus versicolor)*. *Carcinogenesis* 20(8):1637–1640, 1999.

9. Kim, Kacew, Lee.

10. Zhu JS; Halpern G; Jones K: The scientific rediscovery of an ancient Chinese herbal medicine: *Cordyceps sinensis*. Part I. *J Altern Complement Med* 4(3):295, 1998.

11. Shao G; You ZJ; Gu XC; et al.: Treatment of hyperlipidemia with *Cordyceps sinensis*: A double blind placebo control trial. *Int J Orient Med* 15(2):77–80, 1990.

12. Agarwal OP: Prevention of atheromatous heart disease. *Angiology* 36(8):485–492, 1985.

13. Everson GT; Daggy BP; McKinley C; Story JA: Effects of psyllium hydrophilic mucilloid on LDL-cholesterol and bile acid synthesis in hypercholesterolemic men. *J Lipid Res* 33(8):1183–1192, 1992.

14. Gerhardt AL; Gallo NB: Full-fat rice bran and oat bran similarly reduce hypercholesterolemia in humans. *J Nutr* 128(5):865–869, 1998.

15. Lupton JR; Robinson MC; Morin JL: Cholesterol-lowering effect of barley bran flour and oil. *J Am Diet Assoc* 94(1):65–70, 1994.

16. Kabir Y; Kimura S: Dietary mushrooms reduce blood pressure in spontaneously hypertensive rats (SHR). *J Nutr Sci Vitaminol* (Tokyo) 35(1):91–94, 1989.

17. Zhou M; Chen Y; Ouyang Q; et al.: Reduction of the oxidative injury to the rabbits with established atherosclerosis by protein bound polysaccharide from *Coriolus versicolor*. *Am J Chin Med* 28(2):239–249, 2000.

18. Wang J; Lu YC; Zhen EZ; et al.: Effects of lipid peroxides on prostacyclin and thromboxane generation in hypercholesterolemic rabbits. *Exp Mol Pathol* 48(2):153–160, 1988.

19. Veldman FJ; Nair CH; Vorster HH; et al.: Possible mechanisms

through which dietary pectin influences fibrin network architecture in hypercholesterolaemic subjects. *Throm Res* 93(6):253–264, 1999.

20. Shimizu A; Yano T; Saito Y; Inada Y: Isolation of an inhibitor of platelet aggregation from a fungus, *Ganoderma lucidum. Chem Pharm Bull* (Tokyo) 33(7):3012–3015, 1985.

21. Kanmatsuse K; Kajiwara N; Hayashi K; et al.: Studies on *Ganoderma lucidum*. I. Efficacy against hypertension and side effects. *Yakugaku Zasshi* 105(10):942–947, 1985.

22. Adachi K; Nanba H; Otsuka M; Kuroda H: Blood pressure-lowering activity present in the fruit body of *Grifola frondosa* (maitake). I. *Chem Pharm Bull* (Tokyo) 36(3):1000–1006, 1988.

23. Zhu, Halpern, Jones, pp. 294–295.

24. Zhu JS; Halpern G; Jones K: The scientific rediscovery of a precious ancient Chinese herbal regimen: *Cordyceps sinensis*. Part II. *J Altern Complement Med* 4(4):437–438, 1998.

# Glossary

**ACEMANNAN:** A mannose polysaccharide from the *Aloe vera* plant. Also called acetylated polymannans, APM, and polymannose, the compound has wound-healing and immune-modulating properties.

**ACTIVE HEXOSE CORRELATED COMPOUND (AHCC):** A polysaccharide derived from the shiitake mushroom with immune-stimulating and antitumor properties.

**ADHD:** See ATTENTION DEFICIT HYPERACTIVITY DISORDER.

**AHCC:** See ACTIVE HEXOSE CORRELATED COMPOUND.

**AIDS:** Final stage of infection with the HIV virus, which over time compromises the immune system by killing off helper T cells.

**ALBUMIN:** A blood protein manufactured in the liver that prevents plasma loss from the capillaries; low levels cause fluid to accumulate in the abdomen and in the tissues.

**ALZHEIMER'S DISEASE:** A degenerative disease of the brain that results in progressive loss of memory and intellectual capacity.

**AMINO ACIDS:** Organic compounds that are the building blocks of proteins.

**ANGINA:** Severe chest pain caused by insufficient blood flow to the heart muscle from coronary artery disease.

**ANTIBODIES:** Glycoproteins the body produces to neutralize or destroy antigens.

**ANTIGENS:** Any substance, including bacteria, viruses, and transplanted cells or organs, that incites an antibody response.

**ANTIHISTAMINE:** A class of drugs used to treat allergies that block the effects of histamine.

**ANTIOXIDANTS:** Substances that protect cells from free-radical damage or that neutralize free radicals.

**APOPTOSIS:** Programmed cell death, which speeds up in certain illnesses (psoriasis and HIV for example) and slows down in others, cancer being a primary example. Apoptosis is normal, unless it occurs at unusual rates or in unusual ways.

**ARABINOGALACTANS:** Complex polysaccharides found in many fruits and vegetables and constructed from galactose and arabinose, or gum sugars.

**ARABINOSE:** Monosaccharides sometimes called gum sugars.

**ARTERIOSCLEROSIS:** Thickening and hardening of the arteries.

**ASCITES:** A condition in which fluid accumulates in the abdomen, leading to swelling. Normally, albumin, a protein manufactured in the liver, prevents ascites from occurring. Cancer, cirrhosis, and hepatitis are common causes of low albumin levels.

**ATHEROSCLEROSIS:** Cholesterol deposits in the arteries.

**ATTENTION DEFICIT HYPERACTIVITY DISORDER (ADHD):** A condition that affects children and adults, believed to result from a defect in the way the brain handles the neurochemical dopamine, which leads to hyperactivity and learning disorders.

**B CELLS:** Cells that head up the body's humoral immunity, producing the antibodies that float in the blood and neutralize or destroy unwanted particles or organisms.

**BETA-GLUCANS:** Polysaccharides from the cell walls of mushrooms and yeasts, as well as from rice, oat, and barley brans. Beta-glucans have antitumor, antiviral, antibacterial, antifungal, antiparasitic and cholesterol-lowering actions.

**BLOOD-BRAIN BARRIER:** A barrier formed by the blood vessels and outer tissues of the brain that prevents toxins and pathogens from entering the brain and the cerebrospinal fluid.

**BLOOD HYPERCOAGULABILITY:** A condition in which the blood clots too easily, which can potentially lead to heart attacks and strokes unless treated with blood thinners like heparin.

**BLOOD UREA NITROGEN (BUN):** A normal waste product whose levels rise in the blood or serum in kidney disease.

**BOOP:** Short for bronchiolitis obliterans with organizing pneumonia, it's an idiopathic disorder of the lungs with features of viral pneumonia and autoimmune diseases. Scar and inflamed tissue form in the bronchial tubes, so over time they become heavy and stiff, making breathing labored and difficult.

**BOVINE TRACHEAL CARTILAGE:** A polysaccharide from the trachea of cows that has immune-stimulating and antitumor properties.

**BRONCHIOLITIS OBLITERANS WITH ORGANIZING PNEUMONIA:** See BOOP.

**CANCER:** A line of cells that grows without restraint.

**CHITIN:** A polysaccharide that quells allergic reactions; it's found in mushroom cell walls and in the shells of crustaceans, including shrimp, krill, and crabs.

**CHITOSAN:** Chitin modified by acid and alkali. Unlike chitin, chitosan can bind fat and is used in weight-loss supplements.

**CHLAMYDIA PNEUMONIAE:** A mycoplasma that causes pneumonia and has also been linked to heart disease.

**CHRONIC FATIGUE SYNDROME (CFS):** A disease characterized by low-grade fevers, night sweats, swollen lymph nodes, muscle and joint pain, autonomic nervous system abnormalities, short-term memory problems, and exhaustion.

**CHRONIC OBSTRUCTIVE PULMONARY DISEASE (COPD):** Chronically labored and shallow breathing (particularly on exertion) that's characteristic of several chronic lung diseases, including emphysema and asthma.

**COLEY'S TOXINS:** A vaccine devised by Dr. William Coley a hundred years ago to treat sarcomas and other cancers.

**COMPLEMENT:** A group of proteins that directly kills invaders or stimulates antibodies and white blood cells to destroy foreign cells.

**CONDYLOMA:** A sexually transmitted viral disease, better known as venereal warts.

**CONTROL GROUP:** In scientific studies, the group that receives a placebo or that serves as the standard for comparison with the experimental group.

**CORDYCEPS:** A mushroom used in China to treat asthma, hepatitis, low libido, and infertility. A favorite among athletes to boost endurance, the mushroom also crunches free radicals and helps restore immune functioning.

**CORIOLUS VERSICOLOR:** A fibrous, medicinal mushroom used in Japan and China to treat cancer.

**CREATININE:** A waste product in muscle tissue and blood formed by the metabolism of creatine (an organic acid that enables muscles to contract); creatinine levels rise in kidney disease.

**CROHN'S DISEASE:** Chronic inflammation of the colon and ileum.

**CRYPTOSTRONGYLUS PULMONI:** Latin for "hidden lungworm." A newly discovered roundworm implicated as a cause or cofactor in chronic fatigue syndrome.

**CS-4:** An immune-stimulating extract of the cordyceps mushroom.

**CYTOKINE:** Proteins or glycoproteins, including interleukins, tumor necrosis factor, lymphokines, and interferons, which are vital to the immune response and can cause flu-like symptoms as they battle pathogens. More than a hundred cytokines have been discovered.

**DEXA SCAN:** A machine that measures the percentages of body fat and lean tissue; it can also measure bone loss.

**DIABETES:** Diseases that result when the body isn't making enough insulin—a hormone produced by the pancreas to regulate blood sugar—or when the body is insensitive to the insulin being generated.

**DISACCHARIDE:** Two saccharides linked together to form a substance with two molecules.

**DOUBLE-BLIND STUDY:** A scientific study in which neither the researchers nor the patients know who is getting the drug and who is getting the placebo.

**EDEMA:** Excess accumulation of fluid in the tissues, leading to swelling.

**ENZYME:** A protein or glycoprotein that serves as a catalyst for biochemical reactions in the body.

**ERYSIPELAS:** A severe skin infection caused by a strain of strep.

**ESSENTIAL SACCHARIDE:** One of the eight essential sugars the body needs to perform vital immune, neurological, and communications functions. These sugars are mannose, glucose, galactose, xylose, fucose, N-acetylglucosamine, N-acetylgalactosamine, and N-acetylneuraminic acid.

**FETAL ALCOHOL SYNDROME:** A syndrome caused by maternal alcohol abuse in which the newborn exhibits symptoms of alcohol withdrawal and may experience lifelong physical and mental deficits, including short stature, learning disabilities, and hyperactivity.

**FIBROMYALGIA:** A disorder that causes painful trigger points in the muscles that hurt acutely to the touch.

**FIBROSARCOMA:** A sarcoma of the fibrous connective tissue.

**FOAM CELLS:** A macrophage filled with debris and rich in free radicals.

**FREE RADICAL:** A highly reactive atom or atoms that can damage tissues.

**FUCOSE:** One of the eight essential saccharides.

**GAG LAYER:** Short for glycosaminoglycan layer, it's a glycoprotein and the body's mucosal-lining defensive barrier. It binds water very strongly and is largely responsible for us not leaking or emptying out—despite the fact that we're more than 80 percent water. Wherever the barrier is defective, toxins and pathogens can penetrate, causing inflammation and infection.

**GALACTOSE:** One of the eight essential saccharides.

**GANGLIOSIDE:** A covering of nerve and other cells that consists of fats and saccharides.

**GLUCOSAMINE:** A metabolic product of the essential saccharide N-acetylglucosamine.

**GLUCOSE:** One of the eight essential saccharides.

**GLUTATHIONE:** A potent detoxifier composed of three amino acids and concentrated in the liver.

**GLUTATHIONE PEROXIDASE:** The enzyme responsible for generating glutathione, an important antioxidant.

**GLYCOBIOLOGY:** The science that studies the role of sugars in living things.

**GLYCOFORM:** A catch-all term for large molecules made of sugars in combination with proteins and/or fats.

**GLYCOLIPID:** Synonym for liposaccharide, it's a compound consisting of saccharides and fats.

**GLYCONUTRIENTS:** Foods and supplements that contain some or all of the eight essential saccharides.

**GLYCOPROTEIN:** A compound consisting of saccharides and proteins.

**GONG:** Also called kung. A Chinese term that means cultivation, as in personal cultivation. Kung-fu or Gong-fu is a practice in which martial arts proficiency and mastery is built by practicing a set of skills daily in a focused and non-obsessed manner.

**GRAM:** 1,000 milligrams.

**GULF WAR SYNDROME (GWS):** Afflicting an estimated 100,000 men and women who served during the Gulf War, the disease is marked by muscle pain, short-term memory problems, autonomic nervous system disorders, lymph node swelling, sleep disorders, and low-grade fevers.

**HDL:** Short for high-density lipoprotein, it's the so-called good cholesterol.

**HEART FAILURE:** Temporary or chronic, heart failure occurs when the heart fails to maintain adequate blood circulation. Symptoms include swelling (edema), shortness of breath, and bluish discoloration of the skin from poor oxygenation of the blood.

**HELICOBACTER PYLORI:** A bacterium responsible for some kinds of peptic ulcers; it has also been linked to heart disease.

**HELPER T CELLS:** Also called CD4 cells, they are activated in the normal immune response and crippled by the HIV virus.

**HEMOLYTIC-UREMIC SYNDROME:** A serious disease sometimes caused by *E. coli* bacteria that results in platelets and red blood cells clumping together, instigating multiple organ damage and kidney failure.

**HEPATITIS:** Inflammation of the liver caused by viruses, bacteria, parasites, alcohol, poisons and drugs that leads to jaundice and liver enlargement. Hepatitis A, contracted through contaminated water or food, rarely becomes chronic. Hepatitis B (transmitted through sexual contact or blood) and hepatitis C (primarily blood-borne) can become chronic, and lead to liver failure, liver cancer, and cirrhosis.

**HERPES VIRUSES:** A group of viruses, some of which cause blister-like eruptions on the skin or mucous membranes and can be life-threatening in the immunocompromised and newborn.

**HISTAMINE:** A substance released from mast cells as part of the body's immune and allergic response.

**HIV:** The virus that causes AIDS.

**HYPERTENSION:** High blood pressure.

**IGE:** An antibody that's activated in allergic responses and against infestations from parasites.

**IMMUNE SYSTEM:** White blood cells and the chemicals they produce, including cytokines and antibodies, which neutralize and destroy pathogens and fight off disease.

**IMMUNOMODULATOR:** A substance that downregulates when the immune system is overactive and upregulates when the immune system is underactive.

**INTERFERON:** See CYTOKINE.

**INTERLEUKIN:** See CYTOKINE.

**INTERSTITIAL CYSTITIS:** Chronic inflammation of the bladder.

**INULIN:** A polysaccharide found in chicory, onion, garlic, and the dahlia plant that promotes colon health.

**IN VITRO:** In the test tube.

**IN VIVO:** In the organism.

ISABGOL HUSKS: A psyllium fiber that contains polysaccharides.

KAPOSI'S SARCOMA: Common in AIDS patients, Kaposi's sarcoma is a skin cancer identified by telltale bluish-red nodules.

LDL: Short for low-density lipoprotein, it's the so-called bad cholesterol.

LECTIN: A protein molecule that binds or attracts sugars.

LENTINAN: A beta-glucan extract of the shiitake mushroom with immune-stimulating properties.

LING ZHI-8: A glycoprotein extract of the reishi mushroom.

LIPIDS: Fats and triglycerides.

LIPOPEROXIDE: A destructive free radical generated from oxidizing activity on deposited cholesterol.

LIPOSACCHARIDE: Synonym for glycolipid, it's a compound consisting of fats and saccharides.

LUPUS: An autoimmune connective-tissue disease that primarily afflicts women and is characterized by skin lesions, joint pain, arthritis, and kidney disease.

LYMPHOCYTE: A B or T white blood cell.

LYMPHOKINE: See CYTOKINE.

MACROPHAGE: The largest white blood cell in the body, its main function is to ingest and analyze microbes. It also monitors the state of health of other cells and influences healing.

MAITAKE D-FRACTION: An immune-stimulating beta-glucan extract of the maitake mushroom.

MAITAKE MUSHROOM: A mushroom with immune-stimulating and anti-tumor properties.

MALONDIALDEHYDE (MDA): A chemical that is used to track destructive free radicals called lipoperoxides.

MANNOSE: One of the eight essential saccharides.

MAST CELLS: Cells activated in the immune and allergic response that release histamine.

MDA: See MALONDIALDEHYDE.

METASTASIS: The spreading of cancer cells from one part of the body to another.

METASTASIZE: The spreading of cancer cells from one part of the body to another.

MONOSACCHARIDE: One sugar. From monosaccharides, the simplest form of sugar, more complex molecules are assembled.

MULTICELLULAR INTELLIGENCE: The elaborate, elegant communications system of cells that enables us to maintain our identity and structure in the face of free radicals and other degenerative forces.

**MULTIPLE SCLEROSIS:** An autoimmune disease in which the immune system's white cells progressively attack the myelin as if it were foreign.

**MURILL MUSHROOM:** A mushroom with immune-stimulating and anti-tumor properties.

**MUSCARINE:** A toxin found in certain toadstools that induces vomiting, cramps, and diarrhea within a few minutes to a few hours after eating. It can also cause seizures, coma, and death—although full recovery is possible with swift therapy.

**MYCOPLASMA:** A pathogen that shares features of both viruses and bacteria, and which responds to certain antibiotics.

**MYCOPLASMA PNEUMONIAE:** A mycoplasma often found in patients with Gulf War syndrome, chronic fatigue syndrome, and AIDS. It also causes pneumonia in normal individuals, hence its name.

**MYELIN:** The sheaths on nerves that insulate the nerve fibers much like the insulation that covers electrical wires.

**N-ACETYLGALACTOSAMINE:** One of the eight essential saccharides.

**N-ACETYLGLUCOSAMINE:** One of the eight essential saccharides.

**N-ACETYLNEURAMINIC ACID:** One of the eight essential saccharides.

**NATURAL KILLER CELLS:** White blood cells that dissolve pathogens and abnormal or infected cells. Like macrophages, they traverse tissues to guard against invaders and ensure the body's survival.

**NEOPLASM:** A cancer.

**NEUROTRANSMITTER:** A type of chemical that transmits nerve impulses across a synapse.

**NEUTROPHIL:** Also called a pus cell because it releases an enzyme that dissolves cells and causes pus to form, a neutrophil is a white blood cell critical to the immune response.

**OLIGOFRUCTOSE:** Inulin that has been broken down into smaller molecules. The sugar promotes colon health and has been shown to reduce the number of colds in young children.

**OLIGOSACCHARIDE:** Three to six monosaccharides linked together.

**OMEGA 3 FATTY ACID:** An active component of fish oils.

**ONCOGENE:** A gene inserted into normal cells that causes the cells to become cancerous. Oncogenes are often transmitted by viruses.

**OSTEOARTHRITIS:** A disease mostly of older people characterized by chronic degeneration of the joint cartilage.

**PARKINSON'S DISEASE:** A neurological disease characterized by tremors and rigidity that progressively becomes worse as the cells that produce the neurochemical dopamine die off.

PECTIN: A polysaccharide from citrus fruit peel or apple pulp. Rich in the essential saccharide galactose, pectins lower cholesterol in humans and inhibit lung metastases in mice with prostate cancer.

PEMPHIGOID: An autoimmune disease of the skin that results in painful blisters and ulcers.

PHALLODINE POISONING: Caused by the toxic mushroom *Amanita phalloides*, it can result in liver and kidney failure and death.

POLYSACCHARIDE: Many monosaccharides (from hundreds to thousands) linked together. Starch is a polysaccharide, as is glycogen.

POLYSACCHARIDE K: Also called PSK and krestin. A beta-glucan extract from the *Coriolus versicolor* mushroom used to treat cancer in Japan.

POLYSACCHARIDE P: Also called PSP. A beta-glucan extract from the *Coriolus versicolor* mushroom used to treat cancer in China.

PSORIASIS: A disease of the skin that results in inflammation and excessive reproduction of skin cells.

REISHI MUSHROOM: A mushroom that has been shown to be effective against hepatitis and cancers, particularly leukemia and sarcomas, and decreases side effects from radiation. In addition, reishi suppresses herpes viruses and allergic reactions, enhances sleep, reduces the effects of high-altitude sickness, and restores immune functioning.

RHEUMATOID ARTHRITIS: A chronic autoimmune disease that causes joint stiffness, inflammation, and sometimes deformity.

RHINOVIRUS: The virus that causes the common cold.

ROTAVIRUS: A virus that causes severe, dehydrating diarrhea in young children.

SACCHARIDE: *Saccharide, sugar* and *carbohydrate* mean the same thing. *Saccharide* tends to be used more in scientific circles.

SACCHARIDE COMPLEXES: Polysaccharide dietary supplements that contain many or all of the eight essential saccharides.

SARCOMA: A cancer of the connective tissue, including muscle and bone.

SERRATIA MARCESCENS: One of the bacterial components of Coley's toxins.

SHIITAKE MUSHROOM: An immune-stimulating mushroom that also helps lower cholesterol and triglyceride levels.

SJÖGREN'S SYNDROME: An autoimmune disease characterized by dry, irritated mucous membranes, including those in the eyes, nose, mouth, vulva, and vagina.

SOD: See SUPEROXIDE DISMUTASE.

**SUPEROXIDE DISMUTASE (SOD):** A blood enzyme that destroys free radicals.

**SUPPRESSOR T CELL:** This type of T cell, also called a CD8 cell, slows down or stops the immune response after an infection has been eradicated.

**SYNAPSE:** The junction between a nerve cell and the tissue (another nerve or muscle or gland) that it affects.

**TAMOXIFEN:** An estrogen blocker used to treat breast cancer.

**T CELL:** A white blood cell that regulates cellular immunity and neutralizes challenges by identifying, killing, or ingesting pathogens. T cells also play a role in coordinating other immune cells.

**TERATOGEN:** Any substance or process that causes birth defects.

**TERATOLOGY:** The branch of medicine that studies birth defects.

**TETRASACCHARIDE:** Four saccharides linked together.

**TH1 RESPONSE:** A cell-mediated response in which immune cells that directly annihilate pathogens are dominant; certain cytokines predominate as well.

**TH2 RESPONSE:** The body's humoral response, in which B cells produce proteins called antibodies against the invading microbes, the antigens.

**TREHALOSE:** A disaccharide (two sugars) of glucose that prevents osteoporosis in mice.

**TRIGLYCERIDES:** Lipids (fats) composed of fatty acids and glycerol that are transported in the blood by lipoproteins. Triglycerides are the most abundant fat in our diets and bodies and an important source of energy.

**TUMOR NECROSIS FACTOR:** See CYTOKINE.

**ULCERATIVE COLITIS:** Chronic inflammation and ulceration in the colon.

**XENOSUBSTRATE:** A toxin in our environment and food that our bodies were not designed to handle. Xenosubstrates compete with normal substrates—which may be food or other substances in the body—for valuable enzymes.

**XYLOSE:** One of the eight essential saccharides.

# Index

# About the Authors

EMIL I. MONDOA, M.D., developed an interest in the more esoteric aspects of plant sugars when he experienced significant and permanent relief from a stubborn health challenge by supplementing his diet with plant sugars derived from *Aloe vera* and tree gums. To better understand his experience, he set out to uncover what had been published around the world about the role of sugars in the body and the effect of these sugars on cell function and health. He discovered that throughout history, traditional peoples have used sugars derived from plants, fungi, and animals to help the body heal and to improve normal functioning and resistance to stress and disease. He also found substantial validation of these traditional practices by modern scientific research. Certain sugars are essential for the normal functioning of our immune systems and in the remodeling and recovery of all our tissues from stress and daily wear and tear. *Sugars That Heal* is the result of a five-year effort to bring information about this affordable, safe means of preventive health and self-care to the attention of the worldwide public. Dr. Mondoa is currently working to improve communication between scientists and health-care practitioners to increase our understanding of these sugars.

MINDY KITEI is an editor, writer, and instructor who works in Philadelphia. She is a former editor at *TV Guide* and *Philadelphia Magazine* and contributor to TV Guide Online and the *Philadelphia Daily News*. For the Philadelphia arts and lifestyle magazine *Applause*, she served as a health columnist for eight years. She has taught journalism at Temple University and Rosemont College and sits on the board of Scribe Video Center, a multicultural arts organization based in Philadelphia. She holds a B.A. in communications from the University of Pennsylvania, and she received her master's in journalism from the Medill School of Journalism at Northwestern University.